Penguin Health
Freedom and Choice in Childbirth

Sheila Kitzinger, MBE, M.Litt., is a childbirth educator and social anthropologist. After training to teach drama and voice production, she read social anthropology at Oxford University, where she then carried out research on race relations, going on to teach and do research at the University of Edinburgh.

Since 1958 she has been developing her own 'psychosexual approach' to birth and has studied preparation for childbirth and styles of childbearing in cultures as varied as those of the Caribbean, the United States and Africa. In Britain she teaches couples and trains teachers for the National Childbirth Trust, and is on its panel of advisers. She is also a consultant for the International Childbirth Education Association. From 1971 to 1973 she held the Joost de Blank Award for research into the problems facing West Indian mothers in Britain. She has lectured widely in North and South America, Israel, Europe and Australia. She was awarded the MBE in recognition of her services to education for childbirth.

Sheila Kitzinger's other books include *Education and Counselling for Childbirth*, *Women as Mothers*, *The Place of Birth* (edited with Professor John Davis), *Birth at Home*, *Being Born*, *Giving Birth: How it Really Feels*, *Birth over Thirty*, *The New Good Birth Guide*, *Pregnancy and Childbirth*, *The Experience of Childbirth*, *The Experience of Breastfeeding* and *Women's Experience of Sex* (the last five published in Penguin).

She is married to Uwe Kitzinger, President of Templeton College, Oxford. Their home is in Oxfordshire, England, and they have five daughters.

Carolyn Armstrong, the woman in the photograph on the cover, was pregnant with her first baby at the age of 30. She read *Freedom and Choice in Childbirth* and said: 'This book gave me the understanding and confidence I needed to tackle my pregnancy in a positive way.'

She had a long, quite difficult labour, but said: 'Even though it was going on a long time, at no point was I worried or upset. I felt in control.'

SHEILA KITZINGER

FREEDOM AND CHOICE IN CHILDBIRTH

Making Pregnancy Decisions and Birth Plans

PENGUIN BOOKS

PENGUIN BOOKS

Published by the Penguin Group
27 Wrights Lane, London w8 5TZ, England
Viking Penguin Inc., 40 West 23rd Street, New York, New York 10010, USA
Penguin Books Australia Ltd, Ringwood, Victoria, Australia
Penguin Books Canada Ltd, 2801 John Street, Markham, Ontario, Canada L3R 1B4
Penguin Books (NZ) Ltd, 182–190 Wairau Road, Auckland 10, New Zealand

Penguin Books Ltd, Registered Offices: Harmondsworth, Middlesex, England

First published by Viking 1987
Published in Penguin Books 1988

Copyright © Sheila Kitzinger, 1987

Photographs by Nancy Durrell McKenna
Illustrations by David Gifford
All rights reserved

Made and printed in Great Britain by
Richard Clay Ltd, Bungay, Suffolk
Filmset in Monophoto Photina

CONTENTS

ACKNOWLEDGEMENTS

Many friends and colleagues have advised me and stimulated my thinking as I considered the pros and cons of different kinds of care, obstetric intervention and the making of birth plans. I should like to thank especially the many women who have talked to me about their birth experiences and also Dr Michel Odent, Iain Chalmers, FRCOG, Director of the National Perinatal Epidemiology Unit at Oxford, Wendy Savage, FRCOG, Sally Inch, SRN, SCM, Caroline Flint, SRN, SCM, and Chloe Fisher, SRN, SCM. Professor John Edwards enabled me to accompany women through counselling and amniocentesis at the John Radcliffe Hospital, Oxford, and I am very grateful to him for this opportunity. Dr David Banta read through the whole book and made comments and helpful suggestions.

I should also like to thank Janet Balaskas for suggestions about active birth movements included in Chapter 6, Dr Judith Lumley for the idea on which the charts on pregnancy care were based, Penny Simkin for enriching discussion, the concept of the charts on pregnancy discomforts, and questions to ask about pain-relieving drugs, and Dr David Chamberlain for material drawing on research in perinatal psychology, some of which I have used in Chapter 14. The Open University introduced me to the practice of 'learning activities' of a kind which I have woven into the text – so that a woman can test what she is reading against her own experience and use the information which she has been given in order to make active choices between alternatives. The charts in these pages are similar to those I developed when writing these courses and in the text I explore some of the same subjects but in a rather different way. The Open University material takes the form of packs containing work books, audio tapes and video cassettes. These are available from the Open University and full details are listed on page 309.

First Margaret Pearson and later Judith Schroeder have given me skilled and unflappable secretarial help and I'm very grateful for having been able to rely on them.

I also want to thank my daughters for their constructive criticism and for a great deal of lively discussion.

I

CURTAIN UP ON PREGNANCY

This book does not tell you how to have a baby or what you should do in labour. It focuses instead on the range of choices open to you in pregnancy, in the kind of care you have, both then and at the time of birth, and on the changes and challenges of those important nine months. There are obviously physical changes. But there are also emotional changes and changes in relationships with your partner, family, friends and people with whom you work, and there is the developing relationship with those whom you choose to care for you in pregnancy and labour.

Pregnancy does not just happen in the pelvis. It affects your whole self, your self-image as a woman and your sense of worth. It changes, often in subtle ways, the manner in which you see yourself and how other people, both men and women, see you. Being pregnant may enhance and enrich your sense of self. Or you may feel that it has taken something away from you.

The information presented here is offered so that you can examine the alternatives, the pros and cons of different ways of doing things, and decide what meets *your* needs. With this in mind there are suggestions right through the book about action you can take. In each chapter there are special ideas to consider, topics to discuss with other people, issues for you to explore more deeply, or facts you need to unearth about the style of birth possible where you live and the options open to you. And all this is put into an international context, so that whatever country you are in, you can still make a plan of action.

Keeping a diary of your pregnancy will help because you can note down your thoughts about these things and the results of each enquiry. You will have a detailed personal record of your pregnancy, too. So as you go through this book have a notebook or loose-leaf file beside you to jot down your thoughts and the facts you have discovered. The activities that I suggest are intended to help you reflect on the information given, record how you feel and work out your own strategies. They are not tests to see if you have read the material properly or to check your understanding. If you prefer to read the book without doing these activities, simply skip them. Or you may like to come back to them later.

You will also find many quotations from women about how they felt, what they did, how they coped with the reality of their own experiences. Some of these women may be much like you, others very different. What they say is important because a happy birth is not a matter of following a method or obeying a set of rules, like carefully following a knitting pattern or the instructions on using a computer. There is no one right way to have a baby. Our personalities and life-styles are different and no one else should – or can – dictate *your* experience.

Choices about birth are never as simple as selecting a can of beans from a supermarket shelf. They often involve powerful emotions – hope, fear, anger, guilt – to name a few. It is understandable that this should be so because birth is not just a matter of pushing a baby out of your body, a demonstration of bio-mechanics, but concerns fundamental human *values*.

Even when we feel most freedom to make choices, those choices are restricted and shaped by social pressures. New choices close the doors on others. When we get the choice of controlling the number of children we bear by using contraception, in effect we lose the choice to have very large families, and women who do so – at least if they are poor – are labelled social deviants and problem cases. As a technology develops which gives us the choice to screen for imperfections in the fetus, and to abort a fetus which is not up to standard, increasingly women lose the choice to bear handicapped babies.[1] When the choice of having complete anaesthetic pain relief in childbirth is available, pressure is put on women to agree to its use and they lose the choice of labouring without drugs. When all women can choose to give birth in hospital it becomes more and more difficult to make the choice, and to get others to agree to it, to give birth at home.

Choice is not just an individual matter, to do with personal and private decisions. It always takes place in a social context, and it is important that we are aware of the constant pressures on us which define and limit the choices we can make.

Enormous changes have taken place in childbirth over the last half century and women's expectations about the whole experience have altered radically. Take this account of birth written from a woman's point of view in the thirties – and intended to be reassuring to the expectant mother. It starts by telling her: 'The thing to have firmly fixed in your mind . . . is that you are going to be a good girl', and warns her that the way to get the best out of doctors and nurses is to do what she is told. Otherwise she will be ignored and neglected. Nurses, though appearing hard-boiled, are 'as sentimental as nursemaids underneath' and a woman who wants to be treated well should placate them and be a good patient. Then there is a description of what she can expect in labour:

Time passes but she is not aware of it as she lies in 'a merciful stupor, not knowing, not caring . . . conscious, but foggy . . . in pain but it doesn't seem real'. Something jolts her out of peaceful quiescence. She is put on a stretcher and carried to another room but doesn't really know what is happening to her – because everything is completely confused, 'like a nightmare'. All she feels is pain. 'Then a rubber ring is fitted over your face . . . you gulp in great breaths. Pinpricks of light and a grinding noise that goes round in a spiral zooms through your head.' The woman doesn't know how long this goes on, but after a time she opens her eyes to see that there is a nurse in the room. She starts to remember that there was something about a baby – and asks, 'When am I going to have the baby?', and a nurse announces, 'You have a fine son born three hours ago.'

We are no longer prepared to hand over responsibility in quite the same way. And there are issues, over and above relief from pain, which concern us: the quality of relationships with care-givers, the side-effects of drugs, the physical and emotional well-being of the baby, and our own autonomy as women.

Yet these changes have occurred at the same time as the whole of pregnancy has come to be ruled by increasingly elaborate screening procedures, childbirth has been made subject to technological control, and a multiplicity of interventions of different kinds has been introduced in even the most apparently straightforward birth.

Raised consciousness has made us more alert, but has not made the experience any easier, not because of the natural processes with which we have to deal, but because of things done to us by those in charge of childbirth which can still make the whole process a nightmare.

Many women today feel as if they have been sucked on to a conveyor belt and are being processed through pregnancy and birth like cars in a highly mechanized automobile plant. They feel guilty when they do anything which holds up the process: asking questions or daring to be persistent in stating what they want. The message they receive, even though unspoken, is that they are being 'bad patients', are naive and selfish, and, if they reveal concern about anything other than safety, that they do not care about their babies.

This means that pregnancy and birth is fraught with a sense of inadequacy and powerlessness. At the point when they are bringing new life into the world and a tremendous power is released in their bodies, women feel most helpless. They are trapped in a situation outside their control.

Preparing for childbirth used to be seen as a matter of doing exercises, learning what happens, and breathing and relaxing in order to cope with contractions. All that training and the rigorous daily practice turn out to be utterly irrelevant if a woman is confronted with a medical system which takes over her labour and manages it, and obstetricians who are convinced they know what is best for her regardless of her own preferences and what she knows about her body. Effective preparation for childbirth must include learning how to cope with the medical system and knowing how to work in partnership with your doctor and midwife rather than passively receiving care. It is your body and your baby, and, though expert counsel is welcome, the decisions should be yours.

A woman who is expecting a baby is not ill. She is *pregnant*. She is performing a normal physiological function for which her body is beautifully made. But, just as with the intricate processes of digestion and the working of bowels and bladder, with sleep, with breathing and the way the heart beats, fear and anxiety that her body may not work correctly, or that she may be subjected to treatment she does not want, affect the way a woman's uterus functions.

This is why thinking simply in terms of risk is so dangerous. It is a self-fulfilling prophecy: if doctors continually remind a woman of risk factors and all the disasters which may be just round the corner, after a while she is bound to lose confidence in her body and see it as an enemy, rather than something through which she expresses herself in giving birth. Her blood pressure climbs, or contractions are ineffective in opening her cervix, or labour suddenly comes to a full stop – leaving her half dilated, in pain, frightened and exhausted. She then actually *becomes* high-risk and needs the obstetric intervention and strong drugs which she may have been determined to avoid.

One important task of pregnancy is to get in touch with your feelings in order to know what is right for you. Saying how you feel is important, too, when you talk to people who are looking after you. Some women think their doctors are going to let them have what they want because they have a pleasant manner. Later a doctor imposes his will during labour, and they discover they were being 'jollied along' and it was part of a method of managing patients. So it is vital to be open and honest about issues that are important to you and not to be lulled into complacency by a mixture of charm and reassurance.

Few doctors have learnt in medical school how to have an equal relationship with their patients, so they feel they are treading on uncharted territory when they enter this new kind of relationship with a pregnant woman. They are usually anxious about it.

It is, on the whole, simpler for midwives because they are women themselves and they too are in an unequal power relationship with doctors. It is possible for you to have most, or sometimes all, of your care from a midwife rather than an obstetrician, and this is an option which will also be explored in these pages.

A price we pay for the safety of birth today compared with the nineteenth century is that we often lack resources when things go wrong, when a baby is born prematurely, for example, or is sick or handicapped. The most profound shock of all comes when a baby dies. Very few of us get any emotional preparation for that kind of experience.

As you think ahead, it is important to consider alternatives if everything is not straightforward – if you are advised to have labour induced, for instance, if labour proves unexpectedly difficult, or delivery is by forceps or Caesarean section, or if your baby is in intensive care. Women often squash these thoughts because they arouse anxiety. All the same, they tend to cluster in the back of your mind and to loom larger still in the middle of the night.

You may find that talking about these things triggers anxiety in other people, too. Friends and family, even doctors and nurses, often prefer not to discuss these possibilities. Such thoughts are branded as 'unhealthy' and you are urged to think positively. That does not solve the problem. And because this attitude is evasive and denies the strength of what is in your mind, it cheats you of the chance of developing skills to cope in emergency and of working out what you want from other people. A woman who has never allowed herself to imagine that her baby might be stillborn, for example, has no idea of what she would want from those caring for her. Is she going to ask to touch and hold her baby or would she prefer the baby to be whisked away unseen? Does she want time alone with the baby so that she and her partner can grieve together without interruption? Or does she choose to be heavily sedated and left by herself? These are all issues which it is difficult to resolve at the time if you have never thought of the remote possibility of such a thing happening.

But of course, plans are one thing. Reality is another. You can never make a blueprint for labour – or for life! Any plan has to be flexible and in that is its strength. The great branches of an oak tree sway in the wind. They do not meet it with rigid resistance. It is because they are flexible that they do not crack. This is why the emphasis in these pages is on learning as you go, on willingness to reassess what is happening and what you want, and on being flexible.

Before you read on, note down the things which are most important to you about childbirth. Discuss this with your partner or someone else close to you. Bear in mind these priorities as you go through the book.

1   **Working out when your baby will be born.**
If you cut round the dotted line you can move the inner circle to mark the first day of your last period, and from there work out when the baby is due and when you are likely to feel the first movements.

THE EARLY WEEKS

Some women glow from the moment they realize they are pregnant and go right through the nine months feeling radiant. Others have patches with aches and pains when they wonder why they ever got pregnant in the first place. A great many find the first three months especially difficult for two reasons: nausea, often accompanied by vomiting, and extreme tiredness.

Judi enjoyed being pregnant from the beginning and says she was 'tremendously excited. I never really believed I was fertile – that I *could* have a baby. It happened immediately we decided I should come off the Pill and we used condoms for three months so that the hormones were cleared from my system, and then I conceived – just like that! I was happy about being pregnant but it was more than that; my body felt, well, *enhanced*.'

Carol does not feel like that at all. For her those first few weeks, the transition to pregnancy, are really difficult. She says: 'I'm aghast at what I have taken on. There is no going back now. Sometimes I feel the baby is a kind of parasite. Then I am guilty about feeling like that. I have had the most awful nausea and vomiting, not just in the early morning but in the evening too, and I have never been so tired in my life. I have had to reassess myself. I can't go on regardless of my body – that's never happened before.' And she added: 'I suppose I have learnt something from that, but it's frustrating.'

However much you read, plan ahead and want to achieve intellectual control over what is happening, pregnancy and birth are processes which sweep through and take over your body.

If you get morning sickness or feel exhausted in the early weeks you may be wondering whether it is going to continue like this throughout pregnancy and the only thing to do is to stop work and lie in bed. Even if you are feeling fine at the beginning you have to make decisions about whether to keep on working, and if so for how long – and if you give up, whether you can cope without the money. Or you may be thinking of cutting down on or modifying work in some way, if that is possible –

maybe working part time or flexi-time. Then there are all the things you normally take for granted – doing the laundry, cooking and cleaning. You may want someone else to take over some of these things or to talk with your partner about sharing them more equally. If you already have children you will need to decide if you require additional help with them. In making decisions about these things, bear in mind that the greatest stress periods of pregnancy are right at the beginning, when your body is adjusting to its tremendous new task, and in the last 6 to 8 weeks, when you may feel tired and heavy and find ordinary, everyday tasks like cleaning the bath, loading the car with heavy packages from the supermarket, lifting a toddler – and even sitting in one position for any length of time – cause backache or make you feel exhausted.

Even at the beginning of pregnancy, for many women there come times when the pressure of trying to carry on as if nothing has changed can be overwhelming, and you may be frustrated, angry or depressed that you cannot organize and get control over your body and emotions, as you used to before you were pregnant. Some women say that, apart from missing their periods, they wouldn't know they were pregnant, and they can go on just as before. But you cannot bank on this, and there is no virtue in pretending that you feel fine if you don't, and thus denying your body's needs.

A woman who is accustomed to being in charge of her life and being able to plan ahead, without having to think whether her body is going to cooperate, may be shocked by the emotional and physical changes of early pregnancy, especially if she feels extremely tired and has nausea and vomiting which, though often described as 'early morning sickness' can continue on and off through the day and get worse again in the evening.

You may even get a disturbing feeling that your body no longer belongs to you, and at times that you have been invaded by a hostile force. Then, like Carol, you feel guilty that you should have such negative thoughts about the baby inside you. There are often enormous fluctuations in how a pregnant woman feels. One day she wakes up sunny and full of energy, the next under a black cloud and wondering why she ever started this pregnancy.

The first surprise of those early weeks is the way in which, long before anyone can see that you are having a baby, your body is totally involved in producing and protecting this miniature creature which is still no larger than a cotton reel. All this is happening when you have nothing to show for it and are probably busy working, perhaps committed to seeing through important projects in your job.

Even if other people do know you are pregnant, women are having babies all the time and your pregnancy may seem to them a secondary matter compared to coping efficiently with problems at work. There are deadlines to be met, difficulties that need sorting out, work schedules which must be adhered to, which don't change just because you are pregnant. To some colleagues it may seem as if you are making a fuss about nothing. Other women who are secretly envious that you are having a baby may feel this strongly, without being aware of their own jealousy. Once they know you are pregnant, some men start treating you as if you were soft in the head and incapable of making decisions in your work. You may feel as if you have been written off as a responsible colleague. Whatever the attitude of those with whom you work, if you enjoy your job and want to go on with it after the baby is born, or to take it up again when the child is older, you will probably feel you cannot afford to slack off now and need to show that you are good value.

The tiredness common in the early weeks of pregnancy is rarely acknowledged, though probably most women feel it, if only in the evening. It can be so severe that you wonder how you can ever get through a pregnancy that starts like this. It seems logical to consider that if you are exhausted at the beginning, it is going to get worse and worse through the later months. This, however, is not the case. Many women who are weary and lethargic in the first three months or so sparkle with energy in the later months. The final few weeks of pregnancy may prove tiring because you are carrying around such a heavy load, but even that is not like the feeling of being completely drained of energy which is often experienced as a woman's body makes its first huge adjustment to pregnancy.

On the following pages are some things other women say they found helpful to deal with the most common symptoms of early pregnancy. If you are suffering from nausea and vomiting or excessive tiredness, go through the list and see what it would be practical for you to do. The chances are that there is at least something you have not tried yet. Jot down any good ideas in your notebook and keep a record of the results. Allow at least four days of experiment before you assess whether a particular course of action is effective or not.

Nausea and vomiting

- Cut out foods which make you feel queasy; for some it is eggs, milk, meat.
- Vitamin B6 (pyridoxine) – 20 to 30 mg. a day. (Since B6 reduces absorption of zinc, it may be a good idea to take supplementary zinc.)[1]
- Cut out greasy, fried and spicy foods, alcohol, smoking and coffee.
- Carry glucose tablets, crackers or fruit around with you. Have frequent nibbles so that your stomach never gets empty.
- Have a snack in the night so that your blood sugar does not drop low by early morning.
- Sip a milky drink last thing at night.
- Get up in the morning very slowly. First sit up for half an hour, sipping a cup of tea (with lemon if milk upsets you) and eating a slice of toast, and then get out of bed slowly.
- Try a high-carbohydrate diet, e.g., dry toast, honey, banana, baked jacket potato, muesli and other whole-grain breakfast cereals, steamed rice.
- Have wheatgerm dissolved in warm milk, a few teaspoons hourly.
- Try ipecac in capsule form (an old homeopathic remedy).
- Peppermint tea may work for you.
- Sip ginger tea: root ginger boiled in water and strained. Add a little honey to sweeten. Or you may prefer capsules of powdered ginger, obtainable from health food stores. Unlike anti-nausea medications, ginger works not on the central nervous system but in the gastro-intestinal tract itself. Experiment with the amount you need. Between 5 and 15 capsules a day are usually sufficient to keep nausea at bay. Sucking candied ginger may also be effective.
- If you are taking iron tablets, see what happens when you stop. They often cause nausea and vomiting in early pregnancy, when they are rarely needed anyway, but do not upset the digestion in later pregnancy. However, a healthy woman who has a good diet does not need iron or any vitamin supplements in pregnancy, and taking them unnecessarily may actually do harm. You should take iron only if there is a clear and specific indication, such as that you are anaemic when you start your pregnancy.[2]
- Keep away from smoky rooms and smells of cooking.
- If you are nauseous in the evening, rest in a darkened room after

returning from work and get someone else to prepare the evening meal. Get more rest. The more tired you are, the more nauseous you are likely to feel.

- If you are vomiting a great deal, try a mono-diet of one food only which you know you can tolerate, e.g., peeled grapes, small pieces of apple, banana, steamed fish, dry toast and honey or yeast extract, for one day. Then add one other food the next day. If you tolerate that well, introduce one more the following day, and continue until you are on a good mixed diet. Go back to the mono-diet if you start vomiting again. You are unlikely to need to do this for more than two or three weeks.

Nausea and vomiting do not usually last beyond the third month of pregnancy, but occasionally it is a continuing problem right up until the delivery. It can be seriously dehydrating and can make you feel very sick indeed. It is known as 'hyperemesis' and the usual treatment involves admission to hospital. A combination of a mixed diet in which fats are restricted, plenty of fluids (sipped slowly) and the ginger therapy may make this unnecessary.

Tiredness

- Cut housework back to basics and put off until tomorrow anything that does not *have* to be done today.
- Make sure you are getting a nutritious diet with plenty of fresh, raw vegetables, fruit and whole grains.
- Get your partner or a friend to go to the supermarket, do the laundry and cleaning, etc., for a while.
- Have a rest in a darkened room immediately after coming back from work.
- Spend one day a week in bed.
- If you can afford it, go to a hotel for a weekend – or explain the situation to a friend with whom you can stay – and spend most of the time in bed.
- Get regular vigorous exercise in the fresh air.
- Make some time for yourself. One way of doing this is to take up some leisure occupation which allows you to get physical rest. It may be easier to take a rest regularly if your hands and mind are occupied. Patchwork or other sewing, the traditional knitting of

little bootees, catching up with correspondence or other writing, doing drawing or painting, even sorting your photo album, are possibilities.

Bleeding

It is horrifying when you are pregnant to go to the bathroom or undress and see blood coming from your vagina, yet this happens to a great many women who go on to have normal healthy babies. As many as 20 per cent experience some bleeding in early pregnancy.[3] The bleeding is often just a few drops, and after it has stopped you can forget all about it. Sometimes, however, it is heavy, like the second day of a period, or there is continuous spotting which goes on for a week or more. In either of these situations there is a 50 to 60 per cent chance of miscarriage.[4] You can have an ultrasound scan to see if the baby's heart is still beating. If it is, you are very unlikely to miscarry. If it is not, there is nothing you can do about it. There is no evidence that staying in bed, or any other form of treatment, makes miscarriage less likely. On the other hand you may feel that you want to retreat to bed, even if nobody has proved that this is any help. All in all, it is probably best to let your own feelings guide you. If you *do* lose the baby you may need this space to come to terms with and mourn your loss. If you just keep on at work as if nothing were happening you may be denying yourself this emotional refuge and later feel cheated, depressed and also guilty that you did not give more attention to the pregnancy.

Pregnancy gives you a chance to get to know and understand your body better. This is not only a matter of learning how it works, what happens as the uterus enlarges and the baby grows, for example; it also means accepting it in a way you may not have done previously. Perhaps this often happens because pregnancy 'gives permission' to concentrate on your body and its needs and on your feelings about it. With the unfolding of life inside your body, you are able to focus on what is happening and can care for and cherish *yourself*. Most of the time women serve other people's needs. You can grasp the opportunity provided by pregnancy to assess your own needs, and, by being positive and taking action, wherever possible develop a strategy to meet them.

Looking After Yourself

DRUGS AND HEALTH

Cigarettes

The evidence against smoking in pregnancy is overwhelming. If you smoke, the moment when you realize that you are pregnant is a good time to give it up, for your own sake as well as the baby's. Tobacco manufacturers see women as a prime target for their marketing efforts and present cigarettes in terms of 'the new woman' ('You've come a long way Baby'), slimness ('Long and slender, light and mellow'), femininity (in the 1960s a cigarette was advertised as being 'as feminine as the ring you wear'), assertive and liberated ('I made a decision about low tar'; 'I want the best taste I can get') and sexually satisfied and personally fulfilled ('More for that extra measure of satisfaction').

Yet a woman who smokes, whether or not she is pregnant, is gambling with her life and health. For instance, she runs the risk of developing coronary heart disease, especially if she is normally on the contraceptive pill – the US Food and Drugs Administration warns: 'Women who use birth control pills should not smoke' – chronic bronchitis and emphysema. A smoker has twice the chance of getting cancer of the cervix compared with women who have never smoked, and the more she smokes the more she is at risk. In 1980 the US Surgeon General reported a steep rise in smoking-related diseases among women.[1]

If you smoked before you became pregnant, you may have given up already. Many women stop in the first few months. American research shows that almost 75 per cent of women do not smoke during pregnancy.[2] A study commissioned by the Health Education Council in Britain (but unpublished) revealed that 15 per cent of women give up smoking at the beginning of pregnancy. They may be concerned about the effect on the developing baby or simply find that cigarettes make them feel nauseated. But the extra stresses that come with pregnancy make some women want to smoke *more* and they long for a cigarette to relieve tension. This may be particularly the case for a woman who is under pressure from work or family, facing financial or housing problems, or who has conceived by accident and has to decide whether or not to go ahead with an unwanted pregnancy. A woman who is advised to have screening for possible handicap in the baby is also under special stress which may make her want to smoke. This is why it seems not only a counsel of perfection but sometimes downright cruel to tell a woman that she should not smoke during pregnancy. Criticizing a woman for smoking is all too often a matter of blaming the victim.

Yet the facts are clear. Smoking is a threat to your life and health and also to that of your baby. It causes 5 per cent of all stillbirths and neonatal deaths.[3] A smoker runs nearly a 30 per cent greater risk of having a baby who dies at or shortly after birth than a non-smoker. Smoking results in miscarriages (a 70 per cent greater risk than if a woman does not smoke) and premature births (a 36 per cent greater risk). Swedish research reveals that there is also a 50 per cent greater chance that the child of a mother who smokes during pregnancy will develop cancer.[4]

But the greatest risk of all is that of stunting a baby's growth in the uterus (a 98 per cent greater risk), and this slow growth continues even after the child is born.[5] The children of parents who smoke are not only shorter than those of non-smokers but are up to five months behind them in intellectual development.

The effects of smoking are compounded with those of alcohol and poor nutrition. So the woman who drinks and has an inadequate diet as well as smoking runs the greatest risk of all.

When a pregnant woman smokes, carbon dioxide forces oxygen out of her red blood cells and those of her baby and nicotine restricts the blood vessels, including those in the placenta. Not only is there less oxygen in her blood but the passage of blood through the placenta is restricted. Another effect of smoking is that the baby's blood gets sticky and this further slows down the blood flow and deprives the baby of oxygen.[6]

The bad effects of cigarettes are directly related to the quantity smoked.[7] So reducing the number smoked, smoking each cigarette only half way down or rationing yourself to a few a day can make a great difference. If you do decide on this course of action, however, *avoid inhaling more*. The tendency is for a smoker who is trying to cut down the number smoked to increase inhalation, and poisons then remain high in the bloodstream.[8]

Passive smoking – breathing in someone else's smoke – can also affect the baby's growth and cause break-down products of nicotine to appear in the amniotic fluid. It is important that other people in the family do not smoke when in the same room as a pregnant woman; this provides a good opportunity for a father, too, to give up smoking. If you are employed outside the home you should not have to work in a smoke-laden atmosphere and could ask to be transferred to a non-smoking section of an office. Even a fan on a desk can produce a little pocket of relatively fresh air.

Taking action

Here is how some women say they have either cut down on their smoking or stopped completely. Make a note of similar strategies which you want to adopt and add any others of your own.

- Reward yourself by buying something you want, like a new dress, with the money saved from not buying cigarettes.
- If you find that small, immediate rewards work best for you, allow yourself an extra small pleasure every week you go without cigarettes – e.g., meeting a friend for lunch, having a massage, enjoying a long phone call with an old friend.
- Get together with a small group of other people who have decided to give up smoking. Six to eight is about the right number. Or you might want to do it just with one close friend. Arrange to meet regularly to check on progress and give mutual support.
- If you smoke when you are bored, fill that time with something else which will take your mind off cigarettes and keep you busy – e.g., getting the baby's room ready, cooking dishes to put in the freezer for after the baby comes, going for an energetic walk, doing anything which involves your hands and which would make it difficult to smoke at the same time.
- If you smoke when on the phone or when watching TV, keep chewing gum or a bowl of nuts and raisins by the phone or near the TV so that you can nibble them instead.

Alcohol

A great many healthy babies are born to women who enjoy having some alcohol during pregnancy. They may like to drink for social reasons, for the feeling of hospitality or festivity that drinking lends to a gathering, to indicate to colleagues or others that they are now 'off duty', or to express a feeling of community in the family or among friends. Taking alcohol is a social signal which marks the switch from work to leisure activities, relaxation after a task has been completed or a particular stress is over, and which serves symbolically as a kind of gift, the exchange of which cements relationships. This is why when we are accustomed to drinking the decision to give up alcohol during pregnancy can be quite difficult. It marks us off as different from many of our friends as well as making us feel somehow vulnerable, almost as if we were sick.

Yet, though an occasional alcoholic drink may help you relax, it is of no benefit to the baby and may actually be harmful. So there is good reason not to drink during pregnancy, or, at any rate, to limit yourself to the occasional mildly alcoholic drink – a glass of wine perhaps, or sparkling mineral water and wine, half and half.

Any woman who drinks heavily during pregnancy puts her baby at risk of developing the *fetal alcohol syndrome*. Symptoms of FAS are growth retardation, neurological handicap (slow intellectual development or mental retardation) and a facial structure which gives a special look to these children: a small head, thin upper lip and a kind of 'elfin' or 'E.T.' expression. The FAS baby is also more likely than other newborns to suffer from cerebral palsy.[9]

Fortunately not all babies of mothers who drink heavily – even those of alcoholic mothers – suffer in this way, though many may not realize their full potential because of the effect of ethanol on their development in the uterus.

Occasional 'binge' drinking – more than a whole bottle of wine, or four or five stiff drinks, for example, can also be dangerous, even when the mother drinks very little at other times. Not only does she have a hangover, but the baby's development may be hindered. We do not yet know exactly when alcohol does most or least harm, but all the evidence so far available suggests that it is during the period of organogenesis, the first 12 weeks of pregnancy, when the organs of the baby's body are being formed, and also during growth spurts in the development of the brain at the very beginning and the very end of pregnancy that the risk is greatest. It may also be that at these critical periods of pregnancy babies can be affected by very low levels of alcohol. And it may be that some are more readily affected than others. One of the problems is that it cannot yet be said with any certainty that there is a minimum safe level for alcohol, below which it can be shown to have no toxic effects.

It is clear, though, that the risk of harming a baby is related to the amount of alcohol consumed. If you drink less than one ounce (approximately two or three glasses of wine or one or two light cocktails) a day the chance is very small. If you have two thirds of a bottle of wine or three cocktails, one baby in a hundred will be damaged as a result. The woman who has a bottle of wine a day or more than four cocktails has a 19 per cent chance that her baby will be abnormal.[10]

Smoking increases the effect of alcohol abuse. A woman who drinks and smokes runs a four-fold risk that her baby will be stunted in growth while in the uterus.[11]

There seem to be some other risks with alcohol, even in small amounts – a couple of drinks twice a week, for example. One study revealed that a pregnant woman who drinks, even a little, is more likely to have a miscarriage.[12] Another research project which looked at women who had one or two drinks a day found a special risk of late miscarriages (after 12 weeks). The risk increased if a woman smoked as well.[13]

One of the risks in drinking during pregnancy is due to the presence of nitrosamines in most whisky and beer. These, as well as alcohol, can cause birth handicaps. The concentration is higher in beer than in whisky and, of course, beer is usually drunk in larger quantities. Even so, it is probably wise to avoid drinking both whisky and beer during pregnancy, not only because of their alcohol content but because of the damage that could be caused by nitrosamines.

A woman who drinks heavily in pregnancy can quickly 'detoxify' herself if she stops drinking, or even cuts down on it, at any stage during the nine months. An encouraging report from Boston City Hospital showed that when women had counselling and help in order to reduce their drinking, their babies' growth picked up from that point on.[14]

If you drink at all, now is the time to take an overview of your drinking habits. Record in your notebook how many times you drank during the last week. If you can remember, also write down the number of glasses of wine or spirits or cans of beer you had each time. Then think whether you ever drink more than this. When you have done this you will have a rough idea of whether you fall into the category of a light, moderate or heavy drinker. Not more than two, or at the most three, glasses of wine or cans of beer, or one hard drink a day, make you a light drinker. More than this and you come into the category of moderate drinker. Five drinks at any one time mark you as a heavy drinker. If you smoke as well, go up one category. Then you can decide if you want to modify your drinking habits or to abstain for the rest of your pregnancy. If you want to stop all alcohol, there are now alcohol-free wines and cocktails on the market, or you may prefer fruit juices or mineral water with lime or lemon.

Reducing or eliminating alcohol at any time during pregnancy really does make a difference.

A note about X-rays

The dangers of X-rays in pregnancy are well known. They can cause malformation and genetic damage which results in an increased cancer risk for a child, and for the children and grandchildren of an adult who was irradiated as a fetus. X-rays also increase sensitivity to dangerous chemicals. There is no safe threshold for radiation, and therefore no minimum level which is safe for the unborn baby.

If a doctor or dentist advises diagnostic X-rays in pregnancy, check whether these are really necessary, and consider getting a second opinion. X-rays of the pelvis should never be done in the first half of a pregnancy. If you decide to be X-rayed, radiation should be restricted to as small a part of your body as necessary, and if the X-rays do not have to involve the pelvic area you can ask for a protective lead shield over that part of your body.

Medication in pregnancy

A pregnant woman in the United States takes, on average, 11 different kinds of medication (including things like aspirin, indigestion tablets and tranquillizers) between conception and the time when she goes into labour, and has a further seven during childbirth.[15]

For two thirds of these drug ingredients consumed during pregnancy, and for a third of those used in labour, there exist no published reports showing that they are safe for the baby.[16] And of those drugs about which reports *have* been published, more than half contain one or more substances which have been shown to affect the fetus adversely.

A teratogen is any substance capable of interfering with fetal growth or producing malformation. Teratogens are likely to have the most effect during the first 12 weeks of fetal development, when major organs of the body and the skeleton are forming. But subtle effects on the central nervous system may occur at any stage of pregnancy, since a baby's central nervous system goes on developing through pregnancy, birth and the first 18 months of life outside the uterus.

Taking any medication in pregnancy is a matter of weighing up the benefits against possible teratogenic risk. That is an equation that has to be worked out with your doctor, and there is a lot that we still do not know about the risks involved – which include the risk of *not* treating an illness with drugs, as well as the risk of the drugs themselves. Some drugs are obviously useful, and some – even those known to increase the chance of impeded development – may be vitally necessary for chronic conditions such as diabetes, heart disease, epilepsy and asthma.

There may also be over-the-counter drugs which you have never thought of as harmful, or a drug you occasionally take – have around your home for emergencies, for example – which could be hazardous in pregnancy. You often cannot tell whether a drug is dangerous simply by looking at the information with the package. More than two thirds of over-the-counter pharmaceutical products taken by pregnant women contain no reference to their use during pregnancy.[17]

Make a list of medication you sometimes take. The package insert will sometimes give enough information for you to be able to assess whether the drug is suitable for pregnancy. Ask your doctor about any for which you have not got this information. Before you take any medicines, whether prescribed or over-the-counter, ask the following questions:

What does it treat, and how?

Are there other options?

What are the possible side-effects?

Could it affect the baby? If so, is it known how?

If I *don't* have it, how could this affect me?

If I *don't* take it, could this be bad for the baby, and if so how?

If you decide that you do not want to take a particular drug during pregnancy, and you continue to suffer the condition it is designed to treat, talk about this with your doctor, since there may well be an alternative for use in pregnancy.

DRUG	SYMPTOMS TREATED	POSSIBLE EFFECT ON FETUS	ALTERNATIVE
Antacid	Indigestion, heartburn	None, but if drug contains bicarbonate of soda it increases your own fluid retention	Milk of magnesia
Antiemetics	Nausea and vomiting	*May cause abnormalities*	See p. 33
Antihistamines	Nausea and vomiting, hay fever	Can cause abnormalities	See p. 33
Aspirin (acetylsalicylic acid: in many products, e.g. Alka-Seltzer, Anadin; read labels carefully)	Headache, toothache, flu	If taken shortly before birth, may interfere with blood clotting (though it is sometimes prescribed to get a better blood flow through to the baby)	Paracetamol, codeine
Cascara (a laxative)	Constipation	None, but can reduce absorption of vitamins in your own intestinal tract	Fecal softener
Ergotamine	Migraine	Miscarriage	Discuss with your doctor
Metronidazole (Flagyl: an antibiotic)	Vaginal and urethral infections	Can interfere with cell development	"
Tetracycline (an antibiotic)	Infections	Can slow down bone growth and stain yellow first set of teeth	"
Barbiturates (some kinds of sleeping pills)	Insomnia	Can cause severe breathing difficulties in the baby at birth	Practise relaxation after you go to bed, and whenever you wake in the night
Iodides (some cough medicines contain potassium iodide)	Thyroid conditions	Can cause goitre	Discuss with your doctor

			Discuss with your doctor
Monoamine oxidase inhibitors (usually called MOIs)	Depression	Can affect central nervous system (but you must come off MOIs gradually): make baby slow to breath, have poor musculature, spells of not breathing (apnea) and feeding difficulties	
Diazepam (Valium)*	Anxiety	Baby may be slow to breathe at birth, have poor muscle tone, spells of not breathing and feeding difficulties	"
Lithium*	Manic depression	Can interfere with balance of chemicals in body and cause goitre	"
Chlordiazepoxide (Librium)*	Anxiety, depression with agitation, alcoholism	Probably little effect but baby *may* have some breathing difficulties at birth and may be slow to suck	"
Anticoagulants	Thrombosis	Interferes with clotting of baby's blood	One kind of anticoagulant, Heparin, does not cross placenta
Live vaccines	Guard against rubella (German measles), measles, polio and yellow fever	May infect baby	Avoid contact with anyone likely to have any of these diseases

*If you want to come off any of the mood-changing drugs during pregnancy, this is best done gradually, or you may have withdrawal symptoms, including vomiting, stomach cramps, sweating, anxiety, depression and inability to sleep. Ask your doctor for help.

Herbs

Maybe the answer is herbs? Some women prefer to treat themselves with herbal remedies during pregnancy and believe that this is a more natural way of healing.

Curative herbs have been used from time immemorial. In the fifth century BC Hippocrates described 400 such herbs, and a Sumerian document recording a wide variety of medicinal plants survives from 2200 BC. Many herbs are pharmacologically potent and modern drugs have been derived from them, though sometimes to treat conditions other than those for which they have been used traditionally. Approximately 50 per cent of all drugs used in prescriptions are based on herbal remedies. Foxglove leaves, for example, contain the powerful drug digitalis. The leaves of aloe vera are a strong laxative. Aspirin is derived from the willow.

It is sometimes taken for granted that drugs in the form of herbs have more healing properties because they are more natural and that they must be safer than drugs in the form of pills and capsules. In fact many people do not think of them as drugs at all. If you decide to take herbs in their natural form in preference to prescribed drugs you should bear in mind that they are sometimes less effective than pharmaceutical preparations because the quantity and strength of the active principle in them cannot be controlled as they can be in the manufactured product. The maturity of the plant, state of the weather, time of day when it was picked – even the soil in which it was grown – may all affect the concentration of the active principle present. It has been estimated, for example, that when comfrey, the active principle of which is allantoin, is used to fight infection, you may need anything from 8 ounces to 8 pounds of dried leaves in a quart of water to make a mixture which is pharmacologically active.[18]

There are other – more serious – problems with herbs, too. When plants are gathered in the wild, not only may one plant be mistaken for another, resulting in poisoning, but there may be contaminants which themselves have a toxic effect. And even the most efficacious herb, when used unwisely or in an excessive dose, can result in poisoning. Ginseng, for example, which is often advocated for 'female complaints' and in oriental medicine to help adaptation to stress, used long-term is associated with hypertension, difficulty in sleeping, skin rashes and morning diarrhoea. This has been called the 'ginseng abuse syndrome'.[19] Aloe vera can cause cramp, nausea, vomiting and diarrhoea. Its use in pregnancy may lead to miscarriage and has a possible teratogenic effect. Taking lobelia may result in vomiting, a drop in temperature, sweating, paralysis, collapse and coma.

Here are some herbs and other substances which women have told me they have found helpful in pregnancy. Most can be bought as herbal teas in health-food shops. Unless I have specified otherwise, about one teaspoonful of the herb has been used with half a pint of water.

Either the boiling water has been poured on to the herb and it has been left to steep for about 15 minutes, or it has been brought to the boil with the herb in it and the mixture has been removed from the heat as soon as it has come to boiling point and then allowed to steep for about 10 minutes. When roots have been used, the steeping has been much longer – up to an hour.

HERB	USEFUL FOR	HERB	USEFUL FOR
Camomile	Nausea	Garlic	High blood pressure
Spearmint	,,	Nettles	,,
Ginger	,,	Spinach	,,
Wormwood	,,	Meadow-	,,
Raspberry	,,	sweet	
leaves		Rue	,,
Lemon	Heartburn and indigestion	Raspberry	Increased uterine muscle
verbena		leaves: one	tone for effective
Camomile	,,	cup every	contractions in labour
Cinnamon	,,	day from	
Cloves	,,	seventh	
Ginger	,,	month of	
Nutmeg	,,	pregnancy	
Peppermint	,,	Lady's	,,
Caraway	,,	mantle	
Rhubarb	Constipation	Blue	,,
Senna pods	,,	cohash	
Dandelion	,,	Witch	Haemorrhoids; in ice
leaves		hazel	pack for local application
Brewer's	,,	Lady's	Thrush
yeast		mantle	
Garlic	,,	Hawthorn	Difficulty in sleeping
Rosemary	High blood pressure	flowers	
Hawthorn	,,	and fruit	
flowers			
and fruit			

Pregnancy discomforts and what to do about them

For many pregnant women, physical changes result in stresses and strains on the body. These are often called 'the minor discomforts of pregnancy' and are brushed aside as of no importance. When you have nagging backache, throbbing varicose veins, painful haemorrhoids, or feel the baby is dropping out between your legs as you waddle about like a duck-billed platypus, this casual dismissal of what you are enduring can make you feel much worse. But there is usually something you can do to ease these aches and pains.

> Make a note of decisions you have made about drugs in pregnancy and any plans you have for alternative forms of treatment, either with other, safer drugs or by non-pharmaceutical methods. There is more information to help you on the following pages.

DISCOMFORT	WHY	WHAT YOU CAN DO
Need to empty your bladder very often, especially at night	Due to pressure of the uterus on the bladder when the uterus is still low in your pelvis; again when the baby's head has engaged in the pelvis.	Avoid drinking just before you go to bed. Lie down for a while before you go to sleep – can reduce pressure and give you a chance to empty your bladder. Cut out coffee, tea and alcohol, which stimulate urine production. Empty your bladder before you go out.
Indigestion/heartburn (a hot feeling in your chest and throat as a result of bringing up acid from the stomach)	Sometimes due to high levels of progesterone and other hormones which soften the valve at the top of the stomach. Can also be due to the uterus pressing on the digestive organs late in pregnancy. Affected by what and how you eat.	Eat little and often. Eat slowly, chewing everything well. Sip ice-cold milk after food. Do not eat late in the evening. Sleep propped up on lots of pillows or a floor cushion. Reduce or stop taking iron tablets. Avoid greasy foods and fried foods. Do not jump up from the table to dish up. Ask others to clear dishes.
Cramp low in the abdomen or in the groin, on one or both sides	Caused by sudden stretching of the ligaments which link the front of the uterus to either side of the groin and hold up the uterus. It happens especially if you sneeze, cough, laugh or stand up quickly.	Move slowly. Avoid jerky movements and changes of position. If you're about to sneeze or cough, bend forward at the hip before you do.
Aching or steady throbbing between your legs when standing	Due to pressure of the weight of the uterus on the pelvic floor muscles and the softening effect of pregnancy hormones.	Practise pelvic floor exercises (see pp. 59–60) regularly through the day. Sit with legs raised to hip level on a couch or stool whenever you can.
Cramp in legs	Due to metabolic changes resulting in imbalance between calcium and phosphorus.	Before bed, sit on floor and stretch one leg out. Hold toes and press heel down till you feel stretch in calf muscles.

DISCOMFORT	WHY	WHAT YOU CAN DO
Cramp in legs (cont.)		Repeat with other leg. Try more milk in diet or take calcium tablets.
Backache	Primarily due to your posture in response to the growing weight of the uterus. The baby may press against your sacrum, the big bone where your pelvis joins the spine.	Sleep on firm bed, avoid sagging mattress. (Put a board under the mattress or put the mattress on the floor.) Stand straight, tucking in your bottom and avoid hollowing your back. Sit on a straight high chair, tuck a cushion in the small of your back. On long car journeys stop and get out for some exercise every hour. When shifting or lifting heavy objects, bend knees and use the muscles in your legs, not those in your back. Avoid high-heeled shoes, standing or sitting still for a long while (keep on the move).
Difficulty sleeping	Because the baby kicks so much, you need to empty your bladder, or you are in physical discomfort; because of vivid or bad dreams, or anxiety.	Take some vigorous exercise every day. Hot bath before bed, use relaxation techniques, read a boring book, do crossword puzzles, play music. See if lying on your side with a pillow under your upper knee is more comfortable. If you are anxious about the birth, the baby or life afterwards, talk to someone about your worries – e.g., your partner, a friend who understands, your doctor or midwife, your childbirth teacher.

Dizziness when lying on your back (supine hypotension)	Because the weight of the uterus is pressing the main blood vessels in the lower part of the body. This slows down the rate at which the blood returns to the heart and makes your blood pressure too low.	Avoid lying on your back. Have extra pillows at night.
Varicose veins (and aching legs)	Pressure of the uterus on the blood vessels.	Keep moving whenever possible. Rest with your feet up. Wear support tights or stockings. When you get the opportunity, draw circles or the letters of the alphabet with your toes while sitting down. Avoid sitting with knees crossed, or on a chair with the edge pressed against your legs.
Piles (haemorrhoids) and varicose veins of the vulva	Pressure of the uterus on the blood vessels. Made worse by constipation.	Change diet, include plenty of fibre, avoid constipation. Plenty of fluids. Never strain to pass a bowel movement. Ask your doctor for a prescription to soothe them. Try a small peeled clove of garlic eased inside the anus.
Skin changes Particularly dry or greasy skin	Pregnancy hormones	Oil in the bath, rich moisturizer for dry skin, skin cleanser and toner for greasy skin.
Brown patches around eyes, nose or on neck		Avoid sunbathing or use a complete sun block. The patches will disappear after birth.

DISCOMFORT	WHY	WHAT YOU CAN DO
Stretch marks on thighs, buttocks, breasts, abdomen	Pressure from enlarging uterus and breasts and all-round storage of fat.	Special creams are sold. They can help keep your skin supple but the strain is beneath the skin. Will fade to silver streaks after the birth.
Red raised patches ('vascular spiders')		Nothing. Will disappear after birth.
Brown line from navel to pubic hair	Shows where the rectus muscle down the centre of the abdomen has begun to peel open inside so there is more space for the uterus.	Nothing. Will disappear after birth.
Constipation	Sometimes due to hormone changes slowing down intestinal action to allow increased absorption of nutrients and water. Uterus may also press against large intestine. Iron tablets can cause or exacerbate constipation (may also cause diarrhoea). Diet is a crucial factor.	Drink plenty of fluid – 6–8 glasses a day. Eat fibre-rich foods – e.g., wholemeal bread, bran, pulses, raw fruit and vegetables, especially figs, prunes. Liquorice may help. Avoid sugar and refined foods, aspirin and iron pills (or take iron only with food). Get some exercise every day.

It is normal for your vagina to be moist and juicy during pregnancy, but if you have an irritating discharge or one that is yellow or green, this is a sign of infection:

DISCOMFORT	WHY	WHAT YOU CAN DO
Thrush (Candida albicans)	Being 'run down' and under stress; antibiotics; diabetes of pregnancy.	Use pessaries or cream prescribed by doctor. Omit sugar from diet. Avoid wearing tight trousers or pants. Wear cotton pants, not synthetic fabric. Wash daily, but avoid long soaking in a hot bath. Soak in tepid water with half a cup of vinegar in it. Suck yoghurt into a bendy straw and then press yoghurt through straw into vagina.

Trichomonas	Can be acquired from partner by sexual intercourse	Use pessaries or cream prescribed by doctor. You and your partner should take course of antibiotics prescribed by doctor. Get your partner to wear a condom.
Bacteria (chlamydia, gardnarella, gonorrhoea)	Can be acquired from partner by sexual intercourse.	Pessaries or cream for you and antibiotics prescribed by doctor for both partners. Get your partner to wear a condom.
Local irritation or allergy	Synthetic fabrics, vaginal deodorants, contact with rubber condom.	Avoid vaginal contact with rubber, deodorants, talcum powder, strong-smelling soap, bath foam. Wear cotton underclothes.

4

CHOOSING THE RIGHT FOOD

This chapter does not aim to prescribe a diet for pregnancy, but rather to help you look at your nutrition and decide whether it could be improved. There are various ways in which you might do this, and the choice is up to you.

There are nine months – or actually 35 weeks from the time when you first realize that you may be pregnant – in which to nourish the baby inside your body and to build a strong and healthy human being able to cope with all the challenges life presents.

I believe that there are several things wrong with the way in which a good deal of counselling about diet in pregnancy is offered: it is often very dogmatic – implying that a woman must drink two pints of milk a day and have liver three times a week or she is starving her baby. It is also often presented as exclusively of benefit to the unborn baby, not the mother. Yet the right kind of food is as important for her own health as it is for fetal growth and development. She is not merely a passive container for a fetus. Pregnancy makes demands on her whole metabolism and without good food she can get very weary and exhausted. Nevertheless she is supposed to ignore her own preferences and put the right raw materials in so that she will turn out a quality-controlled product at the end of the nine months. It is as if she were a machine to make a baby. If for any reason she does not stick to the rules, she feels guilty. If her baby happens to be premature or handicapped she may even believe that this is all her fault, and that it is a kind of punishment.

That approach to nutrition in pregnancy is dangerous and misleading. It blames the victim and ignores the many genetic and social causes of prematurity and handicap.

The countries with the lowest perinatal mortality rate (deaths of babies between the 28th week of pregnancy and the first week after birth) and the fewest babies born with handicaps are those where there is no poverty and where wealth is shared with greatest equality (Sweden, Finland, Denmark and the Netherlands). A pre-term or low-birth-weight baby may be more the result of socio-economic conditions than of anything an individual woman has the power to control. Many of the things which could make childbirth safer and improve the health of babies entail social and political changes. The gap between the rich and poor needs to be reduced.

In any impoverished society women are the poorest of the poor – and the most badly fed. Custom may add to this malnutrition. In some Asian cultures women are undernourished because they eat only scraps after the men have finished. In the privileged countries of the West, and increasingly in the Third World, the power that food manufacturers and the multinational companies exert over eating habits leads to malnutrition because the nutrients have been removed from processed foods. So prenatal nutrition is not just a personal matter. It is a political issue – for all women everywhere.

What do you and your baby need?

There is no single right diet for pregnancy. Innuit women eat whalemeat and fish, few vegetables and no fruit – and have healthy babies. Many African mothers eat large amounts of grain and vegetable and fruit proteins, but little animal protein – and have healthy babies. In New Guinea insects form an important protein addition to a diet which otherwise is very high in starch – and these mothers have healthy babies, too.

So there is no reason why you should force yourself to eat anything you cannot enjoy. In Western society there are always alternatives which can provide the same food value, though sometimes, if your diet contains no animal products at all, you need to do a bit of juggling to make sure nutrition is balanced.

You will obviously need to bear in mind what you can afford. If you are on a low income, some kinds of high-protein food and, depending where you live, fresh fruit and vegetables out of season may prove expensive. Think in terms of priorities which fit your own life-style so that you can add to, modify or vary your diet to suit your needs in pregnancy.

Pregnancy changes your metabolism so that, even when resting, you are using up more energy. Your whole physical organism adapts to meet new demands which put stress on your cardio-vascular system, affect your breathing, digestion and renal (kidney), adrenal, thyroid and pituitary functions (these are the glands regulating the way your body uses energy). The pituitary gland, for example, gets bigger and produces special preg-

Nourishing Your Unborn Baby

	SPERM AND OVUM MEET	FIRST 3 MONTHS	MIDDLE 3 MONTHS	LAST 3 MONTHS
The baby		Cells differentiate. Heart starts to pump. Organs form and develop.	Cartilage begins to harden into bone. Fetus grows.	Brain cells develop. Nerve fibres become covered in fat (myelinization). Bones harden. Fat builds up under skin. Iron is stored. Carbohydrate is stored in baby's liver and muscles in form of glycogen. Liver functions. Fetus grows.
The placenta		Lining of uterus nourishes developing cell cluster. At 8 weeks placenta starts to function – is fully working by 12 weeks.	Placenta grows, stores nutrients, excretes waste products, keeps pregnancy hormone levels high.	
The mother		Breasts enlarge. Uterus starts to grow. May have nausea. May feel very tired and need extra sleep.	Surge in appetite	Uterus enlarges further. Deep fat is stored for breastfeeding. Calories are stored as energy for labour and after the birth.

The idea for this chart was developed from Phyllis S. Williams, 'Time line for good perinatal nutrition', International Childbirth Education Association. *Sharing*, III: i (1981).

nancy hormones which change the entire hormone balance in your body. Your heart works harder and enlarges. The total volume of respiratory gases inhaled and exhaled increases throughout pregnancy. At the end of pregnancy you are using about 15 per cent more oxygen than you were before you conceived.

With all these changes taking place, it is not surprising that many pregnant women – sometimes even as early as the fourth month – feel dizzy or faint if they go a long time without food, and that those who were happy not to eat breakfast, or often skipped lunch, before they were pregnant, discover that they need some protein to start the morning or have to stop and sit down and eat a high-energy snack at mid-day.

> To work out your nutritional needs, start by looking at what you actually eat at present and at your personal preferences and dislikes. In your notebook jot down everything you ate and drank in the last 24 hours. You can look at this as you read through this chapter and check whether you are getting the nutrients you need. You can then add some foods and perhaps cut down on others. *You do not need to go on a special diet in pregnancy.*
>
> There is one special exception to this: if as a baby you had phenylketonuria (PKU, the metabolic disorder for which a blood check is done on every baby after birth) there is an increased chance of having a baby with a central-nervous-system or heart abnormality if you do not go on a low phenylalamine diet in pregnancy. If you know that you were a PKU baby talk to your doctor about this and seek guidance from a dietician.

It used to be assumed that educated middle-class women automatically ate well. But many restrict their calorie intake in the last three months of pregnancy in order to hold their weight gain. They may cut out or reduce salt because they are told it is bad for them, and some are still prescribed diuretics (pills to increase the flow of urine) to reduce mild oedema (swelling and puffiness caused by water-retention in the tissues). Occasionally they even try to lose weight.[1] *Do not go on a strict slimming diet at any time in pregnancy.* Instead, cut out sugar and reduce fats.

Good nutrition enables your immune system to function effectively so that you can resist infection and cope with some poisons – such as in air and water – which you may not be able to avoid. Absorption of lead, for example, is affected by nutrition. Lead is particularly dangerous if you do not have enough calcium (good sources are milk – whole, skim or buttermilk – and cheese) and iron (green vegetables are an excellent source – e.g., spinach, broccoli, cabbage, Swiss chard, kale, mustard, alfalfa, sprouts, lettuce).

When nutrition is poor, any poisons from the environment also *stay* in the body longer. If you are well nourished you have a defence system to resist the effects of any poison you accidentally absorb.

The simplest way to get good nutrition is to base your diet on whole foods: grains which retain their inner germ and outer husk, fruit including their skins (well washed) when these are edible, and vegetables eaten raw or steamed or boiled in very little water with their skin where possible.

Priority number one is to have plenty of fresh food and avoid highly processed foods. This is not only a matter of choosing raw fruit and vegetables when you can, but also of eating them – wherever possible – within a short time of being gathered. Though this may seem impossible in a city, it is easy to grow parsley and other herbs on a window-sill, and perhaps you can drive out to a farm to buy fresh-picked fruit and vegetables at regular intervals. The foods to avoid or cut down on are refined foods like polished rice and white flour from which much of the goodness has been artificially removed. When you eat bread, pancakes, pasta and cereals, select them in their wholemeal form whenever possible. You can also sprinkle wheatgerm and brewer's yeast over other foods. Wheatgerm can be added when baking and brewer's yeast does not taste too bad in orange juice. Combinations of nuts, grains and beans, peas and lentils make complete proteins.

The basic building blocks of a good diet are protein, carbohydrate and fat. Proteins are essential for your own health, for the baby's growth and for the development of the placenta and maintenance of the amniotic fluid. Protein is stored in the body so that all systems involved in labour can function effectively and after the baby is born you have an ample supply of breastmilk. Protein foods include milk, yoghurt, cheese, meat, fish, eggs, beans, lentils, peas, nuts and tofu (soy-bean curd).

Carbohydrates, together with fats, give energy and assist the storage of protein. Some carbohydrate foods are bread, cereals, pasta, rice, potatoes and bananas. Fats – e.g., butter and oil – offer a transport system for the fat-soluble vitamins A, D, E and K, as well as providing concentrated calories.

Vitamins and minerals are vital constructional materials, sometimes compared to the cement which holds the bricks together.

Vitamins

VITAMIN	WHAT IT DOES FOR YOU AND YOUR BABY	CONTAINED IN
A	Important for the baby's cell, tooth and bone growth. Helps keep your own skin and mucous membranes healthy.	Dandelion greens, sorrel, carrots, parsley, green leafy vegetables, dairy foods, liver.
B complex and folates	Involved in protein synthesis (which makes energy available from food) for the baby and you. B12 helps development of the baby's brain.	Yeast and yeast extract, whole-grain cereals, meat (especially brains, liver, kidneys), eggs, bran, dairy foods, fish, nuts, some green vegetables, dried fruit. If you do not eat any animal products, it is wise to take a supplement of vitamin B12.
C	Protects body cells, maintains connective tissue and helps you both absorb iron.	Red peppers, blackcurrants, parsley, sorrel, green peppers, citrus fruit, tomatoes, potatoes in their skins, watercress.
D	Helps absorption of calcium and phosphorus and enables the baby to develop strong bones and teeth.	Fortified milk, fortified margarine, dairy foods, spinach, parsley, dried figs, almonds, watercress, soy flour, liver, herrings, sardines. Sunlight on the body also forms vitamin D in oils in the skin.
E	Helps growth and maintenance of red blood cells in the baby and you, and the healing of wounds.	Vegetable oils, cereals, meat, eggs, milk, wheatgerm, nuts.

Minerals

MINERAL	WHAT IT DOES FOR YOU AND YOUR BABY	CONTAINED IN
Calcium	Works with vitamin D to build healthy bones and teeth and helps growth and protection of nerves.	Cheese, milk, spinach, parsley, dried figs, nuts, watercress, soy flour, yoghurt, egg yolk.
Iron	Helps form red blood cells which carry oxygen round the body. Needs vitamin C to work efficiently.	Black-strap molasses, liver, lean meat, bran, wheatgerm, parsley, soy flour, dried fruit, millet, egg yolk, prunes, dried peas, beans and lentils.

MINERAL	WHAT IT DOES FOR YOU AND YOUR BABY	CONTAINED IN
Sodium and Potassium	Together regulate body fluids. Sodium is a constituent of amniotic fluid and is needed for the increased blood volume in pregnancy. Over-salting of foods, however, prevents absorption of potassium and can cause high blood pressure.	Black-strap molasses, yeast extract, dried fruit, soy flour, bran, parsley, wheatgerm.
Magnesium	Assists the function of B vitamins and retains potassium in body cells.	Bran, nuts, wheatgerm, soy flour, millet, whole-grain flour, oatmeal.
Phosphorus	Necessary for health of bones and teeth and development of the baby.	Available in a wide range of food. Deficiency is extremely unlikely.
Zinc	May play an important part in the functioning of the reproductive organs. Helps growth of baby. Needed for normal concentrations of vitamin A.	Oysters, red meat, liver, kidneys, whole grains, bran, fibre-rich foods, nuts, cheese.
Iodine	Minute quantities only are necessary for correct functioning of thyroid gland and baby's mental development.	Fish, vegetables grown in iodine-rich soil, agar and carrageen (vegetable gelatine), sea vegetables, iodized salt.

Folate and calcium – your special needs

Folate (one of the B vitamins – see page 45) is the only vitamin, and calcium the only mineral, for which the need as much as doubles during pregnancy.[2] Check through the following list and make sure you have at least one food from it every day:

FOODS RICH IN FOLATE

Yeast or yeast spread (richest of all)
Kidney, liver, brains or sweetbreads
Bran or bran products
Peas and fresh, preferably raw, green leaf vegetables – e.g., endive, broccoli, spinach
Nuts
Whole grains – e.g., whole-grain bread

Then look back at the chart on page 45 and make a similar checklist for daily calcium.

Folate and your baby

When a woman does not have folate in her diet she may run the risk of having a baby with a neural tube defect (anencephaly or spina bifida). A doctor in an area where this handicap was common prescribed B vitamins and folic acid for a group of women who had already had a baby with a neural tube defect. They started taking the supplements at least one month before they began the next pregnancy. Another group of women who had previously had an anencephalic or spina bifida baby did not get these extra vitamins. In the group which had been given the B vitamins very few babies suffered from a neural tube defect. In the unsupplemented group far more had neural tube defects.[3] Even without vitamin supplements, improving maternal nutrition reduces the chance of neural tube defects.[4]

Iron tablets

Many doctors prescribe extra iron routinely in pregnancy. This is because the baby takes iron from you to form its own red blood cells. Iron tablets can cause indigestion and constipation and make nausea and vomiting much worse. There is no need to take extra iron in the first three months anyway, because extra demands are not yet being made and you are saving iron by not menstruating. If you find that supplementary iron is causing indigestion or making you constipated, go back to your doctor. Your haemoglobin (red blood cell) level should not fall below 11 (written on your notes as 11g/dl), but there is a normal 7 to 12 per cent fall in blood haemoglobin by about the 30th week of pregnancy, as the volume of blood increases.[5]

How much protein, how much salt?

Poor nutrition is associated with the rise in blood pressure, albumin (protein) in the urine and excessive oedema (retention of fluid in body tissues) which are together called pre-eclamptic toxaemia (PET for short). A pre-eclamptic woman often feels well, but the placenta may function less efficiently and fetal growth slow down, so that the baby is of low birth-weight. Pre-eclampsia and fetal growth retardation are most likely to happen in the last few months of pregnancy. The doctor usually orders bed rest. Induction of labour may be recommended.

Some kinds of pre-eclampsia can be dangerous for the mother as well as the baby. In serious cases she becomes eclamptic. The signs of impending eclampsia are severe and persistent headaches, flashes or spots in front of the eyes, nausea and vomiting, and extreme agitation. Her blood pressure shoots up and she starts to have convulsions. Medical help should be sought immediately if any of these symptoms are experienced.

One well-known study claims that PET is always the result of malnutrition.[6] Whether or not this is so, even in affluent nations poverty, hunger and eating junk food cause reproductive problems, including prematurity and stillbirth. Some of this malnutrition is actually iatrogenic (produced by doctors) – the result of medical advice to eat less given to some pregnant patients.

Weight-reducing or weight-holding diets, sometimes with diuretics ('water pills') to get rid of excess fluids, are still advocated by some doctors in order to prevent or treat PET. They don't succeed in bringing down blood pressure or preventing protein in the urine. An overview of nine randomized trials of diuretics reveals that in almost half the cases reported they did not reduce pre-eclampsia or the number of stillbirths. Fortunately, neither was there evidence of any severe side-effects of diuretic treatment.[7] There are many questions about PET that remain unanswered and need to be explored.

Since protein deficiency is thought to affect the birth-weight, a number of studies have investigated the effect of giving mothers protein supplements in pregnancy. One of these studies, carried out in Guatemala, where there is great poverty and hunger, showed that protein supplements produced bigger and healthier babies. Another research project in Harlem, New York, found, however, that protein supplements had very little effect.[8]

One problem with dishing out vitamin pills or protein supplements is that researchers often do not find out what the women they are studying usually eat. This happened with another research project which entailed giving Asian women in an English Midlands city extra protein and other supplements during pregnancy. Though extra protein made the women put on more weight, it had no effect on their babies' birth-weights. The researchers commented that if they had provided supplements only for those women who were underfed they might have learned more from the project.[9] So they did another study, providing supplements only for those women who were obviously not well nourished. This time they found that extra protein did produce bigger babies.[10]

Protein deficiency stunts the baby's growth. But having *more* than you need is of no benefit to the baby. Two helpings daily selected from among the following foods will meet this protein need: milk and dairy products, eggs, meat, fish, whole-grain cereals, pulses (e.g., peas, lentils, beans) and protein-rich vegetables (e.g., potatoes, cabbage, broccoli).

Nearly all processed foods are highly salted, and intake is increased still more when salt is added at the table too. Excess salt overloads the renal system and causes high blood pressure. There is a strong case to be made for reducing salt consumption, whether or not you are pregnant. Salt occurs naturally in many foods, so with a good mixed diet you are very unlikely to go short of it.

When you are pregnant you may find you like salty, spicy, strongly flavoured foods, especially in the first months. This may be because there is an increased need for salt at that time to form the amniotic fluid. Provided that you have not developed a taste for over-salted food before pregnancy, your personal preferences are the best guide. If you concentrate on natural whole-foods, rather than processed products, you are unlikely to have too much salt. Onions, garlic, lemon juice, herbs and spices, and roasted seeds and nuts all enhance flavour as well as adding trace minerals and other valuable nutrients.

What do you eat?

A few pages back I suggested that you made some notes about what you ate yesterday. Look at these now and check whether your diet had the nutrients your pregnant body needed. Could you have improved your nutrition? Here is what some women discovered:

Clare, in England, is in public relations and has been trying to lose weight:

Morning	Lunch	Evening
Coffee	Cottage cheese and crispbread	Chinese take-away: spare ribs
Coffee	Lettuce and tomato salad	and spring rolls
	Coffee	Diet Cola
	Chocolate bar 'because I was so hungry'	Peanut butter and enriched white bread
		2 glasses skim milk: 'I couldn't sleep. I was hungry.'

Clare's diet is short of B vitamins and protein, though her appetite led her to have some unplanned food after she had gone to bed which partly made up for this, since peanut butter contains both protein and B vitamins and enriched bread has B vitamins too. But she needs whole-grain bread and other whole-grain cereals such as brown rice, and should add dark green vegetables to her diet for extra iron, magnesium, vitamin A, and B vitamins including folic acid. She could get more protein from fresh fish, which would provide her with zinc and iodine as well. In spite of the salad at lunch, she is short on vitamin C. If she had some potato and added citrus fruits, berries and more green vegetables to her diet, not only would her nutrition be much better balanced but she wouldn't feel so hungry.

Sherry, in the USA, has a child aged 14 months, is alone with the baby most of the day and has an evening meal with her husband:

Morning	Lunch	Evening
Prune juice	Rest of baby's cereal and	Chicken, broccoli, squash,
Muffin	mashed beets	whipped potatoes
	Hamburger	Bought fruit pie
	Scoop of ice-cream	Milk drink
	Tea	

Though Sherry has vegetables in the evening and finishes up the baby's beets mid-day, she is short on vitamin C and would do better with some raw fruit and vegetables at each meal. A fresh fruit salad would be better than the fruit pie. Some citrus juice, an orange or grapefruit, straw-berries or melon would be a good idea at both breakfast and lunch, and she could add tomatoes, watercress or celery to the mid-day meal. Since she needs a lot of energy to cope with her 14-month-old, starting the day with more protein at breakfast would help – perhaps two boiled or scrambled eggs and a helping of yoghurt, or a Dutch-style breakfast with cheese. A good high-protein, high-energy snack to keep her going in the later afternoon, when she says she gets very tired, would be a handful of nuts and raisins.

Kerstin, in Scandinavia, is a vegetarian:

Morning	Lunch	Evening
Fresh orange juice	Lentil soup	Vegetable curry with onions,
Whole-grain cereal	Yoghurt	turnips, spinach and brown
with dried fruits	Brewer's yeast	rice
		Side salad
		Soy milk whisked with banana
		and molasses

Kerstin's diet is high in most vitamins and minerals because of the variety of fresh and cooked vegetables, but unless she is getting sunlight on her skin she is short of vitamin D, and it would help if she had fortified margarine or milk, or took a vitamin A and D supplement. If she chooses the supplement, dosage ought to be carefully controlled because these vitamins are toxic to the fetus in excessive quantities.

It is all very well working out a balanced diet when you shop and cook for yourself. It's another matter when you have to eat at your place of work in a cafeteria or restaurant. Here is a self-service café. Starting at the left-hand side with your tray, work your way along, putting a circle around dishes that you would choose:

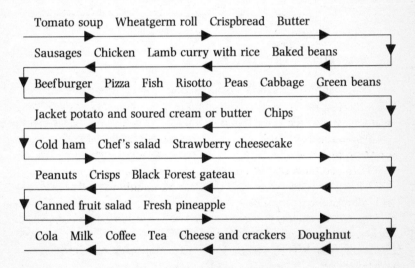

Tomato soup   Wheatgerm roll   Crispbread   Butter

Sausages   Chicken   Lamb curry with rice   Baked beans

Beefburger   Pizza   Fish   Risotto   Peas   Cabbage   Green beans

Jacket potato and soured cream or butter   Chips

Cold ham   Chef's salad   Strawberry cheesecake

Peanuts   Crisps   Black Forest gateau

Canned fruit salad   Fresh pineapple

Cola   Milk   Coffee   Tea   Cheese and crackers   Doughnut

When you have done this, write down in your notebook the things you have on your tray. Then check whether you have the following protein foods and vitamins B and C. You have protein if you chose a meat, fish or egg dish, cheese, baked beans or milk. Vitamin B is in the whole-grain roll, milk, meat, beans and peas, leafy green vegetables (perhaps in the salad?) and peanuts. In most cafeterias food is kept hanging around so that it loses vitamin C. Even so, you will gain some vitamin C if you choose the salad, baked potato or fresh fruit. The cooked vegetables may have been over-cooked and exposed to the air, so you can't rely on them for vitamin C.

The cheesecake, gateau, canned fruit and doughnut are all high in sugar. There is often hidden sugar in commercial soups and other canned and processsed foods. Sugar occurs naturally in fruits and some vegetables, and when you take extra sugar in soft drinks or added to tea and coffee, and in the form of desserts and baked goods, this often overloads the system and feeds you only empty calories. The effect is even worse than that, since concentrated sugar actually draws on stores of vitamins and minerals, especially the B vitamins. If you discover that your meal was lacking in important nutrients or that you were filling up with empty calories, think of some snack foods you could take to work with you to supplement your diet.

At the supermarket

Most 'convenience' and 'instant' products are deficient in vitamins B and C and in minerals. Some B vitamins are eliminated entirely from sausages, processed meat and milk products – processed cheese, ice-cream and commercial yoghurt, for example. Even if you have a large proportion of protein in your diet, you are not necessarily eating the right *kinds* of protein, for the more protein you have, the more B vitamins you require. If you rely on sausages and processed cheese as main sources of protein you may not be getting enough.

Moreover, highly processed foods such as packaged desserts, cakes and biscuits, sausages and other convenience foods 'steal' nutrients from other foods. Whole-foods contain vitamins and minerals which enable you to make use of all the nutrients in them. But junk food leaches vitamins and minerals from your body's stores. Highly processed and refined foods are also very low in fibre and high in calories, so there is a temptation to eat too much of them.

Processed and packaged foods on supermarket shelves often have extra sugar and fat and special additives to preserve and colour them and give a pleasing texture. Red dye No. 2, though banned in France and Eastern Europe because it is believed to cause birth defects, is used in other places in some jams, jelly, sausages, canned food and soft drinks. By law, packaged foods have to be labelled with their ingredients. The first item on that list tells you what there is most of inside the package in terms of weight, and the final one is the lightest part of the contents. But even a speck of a poisonous substance may be harmful, so you cannot go by weight alone.

It is worth reading the labels on all packaged and processed foods. Artificial colourings and sodium nitrite are ones to avoid, together with excessive amounts of sugar and fat. Coca-Cola is composed of caffeine, synthetic colouring, sugar, phosphoric acid, flavouring and carbonated water. Many breakfast cereals contain a high quantity of sugar and are artificially coloured. Sodium nitrite makes processed meat keep its pink colour. It is added to bacon, Spam, beef hot dogs, sliced ham, salami, roast ham and Bologna and liver sausage.

Nutrition in Practice

So much for what we *should* eat. But convenience, the need for speed, the cost of many high-quality foods, and the food preferences of a partner or of other members of the family, all play a part in dictating what we actually eat. Children often have very strong likes and dislikes. If you already have a family, you may plan to have salads, only to discover that they want chips with everything. Then it becomes important to think how you are going to introduce foods, or more of them, which you know are healthy for you in pregnancy in such a way that the rest of the family can enjoy them too. But sometimes, as a last resort, a pregnant woman needs to have her own nutrition plan and eat foods different from her partner's or those of the rest of the family.

The cost of some foods may be daunting. Out-of-season fruits and vegetables are expensive, and because carbohydrate foods are cheaper than high-protein foods you may feel guilty and self-indulgent if you spend money on the more expensive protein foods. On the other hand, there is no need to choose expensive cuts of meat, and there are many sources of protein in vegetables, pulses and grains which, together with cheese, eggs, milk, fish or a little meat, make appetizing dishes. A good vegetarian cookery book will help you plan meals that are nutritious and can give ideas about how to make use of other sources of protein.

The appearance of food on a plate, or different foods to be eaten together, can be a help – and colour especially is useful. Have something white or brown, something green and something yellow, orange or red at every meal. It will look much more appetizing than, for example, chicken, rice and potato purée, and will be a better-balanced meal.

Bearing in mind your own eating habits and what you have noted down about the food you ate yesterday, decide what, if any, changes you want to make in your diet in order to have really good nutrition in pregnancy. You are probably more likely to make changes like this if you limit them, at first anyway, to just two or three decisions which build into a realistic plan.

5

EXERCISE

You may be wondering what exercise you should be having in pregnancy and whether there is any that is best avoided altogether. If you are accustomed to a daily jog or run, for example, or enjoy a friendly game of tennis, or horse-riding, you may be uncertain whether you should stop immediately you learn you are pregnant, whether you can continue right through pregnancy, or whether there is a special time when it is wise to avoid this activity. Even if exercise in general is not harmful, you may question whether certain movements can be risky.

There is, in fact, no systematic medical information to guide you about this. It is a matter of common sense and, above all, your own feelings. *You are the expert about your body, in pregnancy as at other times, and only you can really judge what makes you feel good and what is a strain.* That is the litmus test. Exercise which brings a glow of well-being is bound to be good for both you and your baby – and this applies right through pregnancy.

Major benefits of energetic physical activity in pregnancy are that it tones up your muscles, improves circulation, helps balance and physical coordination as you change shape, and makes you feel good and look good. Movements specially adapted to pregnancy, which you can learn at childbirth classes, help avert aches and pains as you get heavier and enable your body to work efficiently so that you avoid some of the things that can make pregnancy a misery – like constipation and haemorrhoids, accidentally wetting your pants, indigestion, and difficulty in getting off to sleep or staying asleep. Exercise throughout pregnancy also means that you are more likely to feel fit and energetic after the birth and to recover your figure more quickly.

Physical activity has other advantages too. Exercise done for pleasure stimulates the production of hormones called endorphins which are natural pain-killers related to morphine. As you jog, for example, the endorphin level in your blood may rise by as much as 60 per cent. At the same time there is an increase in prolactin of about 40 per cent. This is the hormone which stimulates the breasts to make milk. In animals it is a powerful trigger for nurturing behaviour.

To get a release of endorphins and prolactin you need to 'stretch' yourself. A stroll around the shops will not achieve it. Endorphins are liberated as a result of *stress*. Endorphins are produced in labour too. They contribute to the sense of deep satisfaction which many women experience with the hard work of childbirth.

So regular exercise which you really enjoy during pregnancy tones your muscles, encourages good posture and body mechanics and complete breathing, stimulates an efficient blood flow to the baby, and produces the prolactin which you will need for breastfeeding. It gets you in good condition to get your figure back after the baby is born. And if you start labour with your endorphin level already high from energetic activity it may reduce the pain you experience. When you have enjoyed coordinated physical movements throughout pregnancy this is also likely to have been a good preparation for you to work *with* your body and with the power of your uterus as contractions follow one another like great waves in a strong sea.

Here are some simple and straightforward guidelines about exercise in pregnancy:

You should enjoy it! There is no need to push yourself into doing exercise which you do not like. If a particular kind of exercise proves wearisome and becomes a chore, your body is probably trying to tell you to stop.

It should be rhythmic. During pregnancy hormones are liberated in your bloodstream which soften tissues and make the connecting ligaments between bones more flexible. The research on this was originally done on guinea-pigs, who apparently become very supple when pregnant. For some time it was not known whether a similar process occurred in human beings. But now research shows that it does. This softening process prepares your body for birth so that the bony pelvis has extra 'give' and the cervix and vagina open easily. This means, however, that it is possible to overstretch ligaments which are already very flexible, especially those of the pelvis, and in particular in the small of your back. Bad backache after any exercise which involves vigorous movement – anything which entails hollowing your lower back for example – could mean that you are stretching these ligaments too much. If you keep to smoother, rhythmic, dance-like movements this is much less likely to happen.

It should be non-competitive. Being paced by someone else or trying to surpass their performance could be harmful, because you are likely to lose touch with the messages your body is giving you. A woman who is highly motivated to get herself in shape during pregnancy and remain active and energetic may be particularly at risk of overdoing exercise in this way. Though it is good to know what you want and prepare yourself actively to be in the best condition during pregnancy and ready to meet the challenge of labour, if you know that you have an obsessional personality and tend to tackle things with tremendous energy, you will be aware that your very determination may itself prove a handicap if it drives you to demand too much of yourself. It is important to 'listen' to your body in both pregnancy and labour. You are not taking an exam which has to be passed and you do not need to prove yourself as a woman.

Start any new form of exercise gradually. Tone your muscles step by step and learn how to perform movements smoothly instead of straining. Begin on a new movement or position for a short time only and then lengthen the time you do it or increase the number of repetitions.

Energetic activity should be interspersed with a regular break for relaxation. Release from tension and muscular relaxation is as vital as exercise. Exercise works best for you and for the baby inside you when it is partnered with refreshing rest periods, even if they last only a few minutes each.

As your uterus enlarges you may notice that you tend to breathe more quickly. You also take in and breathe out a larger quantity of air and this enables more oxygen to reach the baby. Your heart beats faster even when you are resting, going up from about 70 to about 85 beats a minute. Heart and blood-flow changes mean that you get a reduced blood flow to your uterus and placenta *during* exercise but increased blood flow – 'flush back' – afterwards. So short bouts of energetic exercise are much better than prolonged ones. Every time you take a rest the flow of oxygenated blood to the baby is increased.[1]

Exercise should not leave you feeling exhausted and washed out. Your own feelings about any activity are the best guide. If you don't feel good after exercise, maybe you are going at it too strenuously. Maybe those particular movements are wrong for you at this stage of your pregnancy. Trust your body. After each exercise session take a little time to tune in to how you feel. For this reason brief regular sessions are much better than a weekly work-out. If you are in pain after any activity, stop it and, if you can, lie down for at least 20 minutes. Then choose an activity which involves different muscles from those you have been using before. There is a lot of exercise in housework. If you have been cleaning windows or hanging washing on a clothes line, for example, both of which entail stretching, get down on hands and knees and wipe the kitchen floor, so that you take the weight of the baby off your spine and flex your arms and legs.

Some women notice that they get contractions when overtired or under stress. Occasionally, exercising because you think you *ought to*, rather than because it feels good, steps up these Braxton Hicks contractions until they become quite painful. Even walking, if done strenuously, does this sometimes in pregnancy. It is a sign that you need to have a rest or change your activity.

Swimming is marvellous in late pregnancy because the water takes some of the weight of your body, and even if you feel rather like a stranded whale on dry land, in water you can move almost effortlessly and feel light and graceful.

Do not hold your breath when exercising. The baby depends on you for oxygen. Any movement which makes you stop breathing is too stressful and should be abandoned or modified so that it is easier. One advantage of vigorous exercise is that it helps you to breathe fully, using all your lungs instead of merely the top part. But if an exercise results in breath-holding it defeats the object. When the breath is held the diaphragm is fixed. If at the same time you are exerting effort, the return of oxygen to your heart may be impeded and you may feel sick and dizzy. This is why energetic aerobics or work-outs on exercise machines are not a good idea.

The balance of gases in your blood could also be affected by scuba-diving,[2] so it is probably unwise to dive in pregnancy. If you are keen to go on diving, restrict dives to 30 feet.[3] One study has shown that more babies with abnormalities are born to mothers who continue, especially with deep dives.[4] Many women get a stuffy nose and congested sinuses in pregnancy because there is an increased blood supply to mucous membranes throughout the body. For this reason deep dives can sometimes also cause burst ear-drums.

Exercise should take place in air which is as clean as possible. Avoid exercising in smog, smoke fumes or chemically polluted air. Jogging by busy roads forces polluted air into your lungs, and though the placenta can filter out some of the toxic elements, it is unable to detoxify your bloodstream completely. When you can, take exercise in the countryside or a park or by the sea.

Special exercises for pregnancy

Exercise should tone the muscles which work to carry the extra weight of the enlarged uterus and the baby – your legs, lower back, abdominal muscles and feet, for example. Sometimes an exercise does nothing to help the efficiency of these muscles. Bending straight-legged to touch your toes is one such exercise. Some movements, such as lying on the floor and raising straight legs off the ground, put strain on muscles which are already under stress, and pain or discomfort can guide you to know when this happens. The muscles most affected by pregnancy are those of the abdominal wall, the pelvic floor – which supports all your pelvic organs – and your back, especially your lower back. Supported squatting and doing gentle pelvic movements on all fours help to strengthen lower back muscles and ease backache. But an exercise which is often taught in birth classes, involving a pelvic rock on hands and knees, humping the lower back and then swinging it down so that it is hollowed, strains the muscles and can make back pain worse. This exercise is fine if you remember always to keep your lower back *flat* as you swing down from the humped position. A good exercise for firming the abdominal muscles is to sit – either on a chair or on the floor – with your hands on your abdomen, breathe in slowly, letting your abdomen bulge out, and then give a long breath out, pulling in your abdominal muscles more and more as you do so. Sit-ups and lying on your back lifting a leg straight up in the air, though intended to strengthen the abdominal muscles, often have the opposite effect. In pregnancy the rectus muscle down the middle of your abdomen, which you may see as a dark line from your navel to your pubis, is under stress. Anything which puts excessive strain on this muscle can make it literally fall apart. The longitudinal bands of muscle fibre separate like a zip fastener unzipping. It can be difficult to regain tone in this muscle after childbirth, and then this must be done very gradually, starting with the breathing movement I have just described and progressing to more difficult exercises.

It is important to exercise invisible muscles, not only those you can see. Pelvic floor muscles which surround your vagina and anus and form thick layers of muscle fibres further up inside, around your vagina and supporting your uterus and bladder, open up as the baby is squeezed down between them to be born. They need to be well toned to cope with the extra weight of pregnancy and be completely released for the birth itself. So awareness of this part of your body and knowing how to contract and relax these muscles at will enables you to have good internal posture during and after pregnancy and also helps you open up to give birth.

The Lift Exercise can be done at any time during the day and it is best to link it with often repeated activities like sitting in the car waiting for lights to change, going up or down in a lift or walking up and down the stairs. Imagine that the circle of muscles around your vagina and your urethra at the front, which swirl round to form another circle around your anus, are like a lift inside you which can go up five storeys. Tighten the muscles first as if the lift is going up one floor. Hold the contraction firmly. Then tighten further as you ascend to the next floor. Hold. Then gradually release the contraction and go down gently and deliberately. Do not let the lift shoot to the bottom. When you reach the ground floor, go further down to the basement by bulging the muscles downwards. (This is what you do when you push your baby out.) Then go *up again* one floor so that you finish the exercise with the muscles well toned. Repeat two or three times. If either during pregnancy or after the birth you find yourself wetting your pants when you laugh or sneeze – a common experience – this exercise, performed so that you act the upward movement of the lift only, will help tone your muscles.

Choosing the exercise that suits you

Now think what physical activities you already enjoy and list them in your notebook. Are there any others you would like to take up which might meet your body's needs in pregnancy? Add these to the list as well.

Ros is three months pregnant and her list was:

> Swimming
> Walking
> Exercise class
> Horse-riding
> Cycling

She decided to find out from her exercise teacher whether she did special classes for pregnancy or, if she didn't, whether she was able to adapt the standard movements to suit a pregnant woman. Exercises were usually done to rather fast music and Ros found keeping up with the brisk tempo tiring, so she was going to discuss this with her teacher too. Walking would be very good, and there were special swimming movement classes for pregnancy at a nearby pool. She would keep up cycling, though a friend who cycled throughout her pregnancy advised her that as she got bigger an old-fashioned, upright saddle would be much more comfortable than leaning forward on to the handlebars. She couldn't arrive at a definite decision about riding, though she did not want to jump in case she was thrown. She was going to see how she felt, and make sure that she always had a well-schooled horse.

Shirley made out her list as:

> Yoga
> Dance
> Aerobics
> Running
> Skiing

She thought the dancing might not be a good idea since they usually danced in smoky rooms where everyone was drinking pretty heavily too. She found an aerobics class for pregnancy and after searching around also discovered a special yoga class. She had been running every morning before breakfast for a year or more and while she was feeling so fit she would keep this up, perhaps slowing down to a jog. She would be guided by how her body felt as pregnancy went on.

In your notebook jot down your plan of action for the exercise you have chosen – how to contact people who can help or join you and any information you need to get.

Many women are now choosing to attend special exercise classes for pregnancy. They do this in addition to classes for childbirth, though there is often an overlap between the two. Sometimes they involve dance. In ancient Greece dance formed a central theme in the worship of Cybele, goddess of birth and of the Moon, and later Artemis, goddess of birth and of all perilous passages. The pelvic rocking and circling movements a labouring woman and the other women attending her made in childbirth were not only of practical help; they had deep religious significance and expressed through each human birth the power of the great Mother Goddess. These same pelvic movements, forming what we know today as belly dancing, have also been used in childbirth and preparation for it among women in Egypt and other parts of North Africa, and are often still used today.

Yoga forms the basis of other exercise classes for pregnancy and includes exercises in deep breathing. In yoga breathing and posture, breathing and movement, are united. It is a way of learning not only how to discipline your body, but also to trust it. It demands serenity, flexibility and balance, rather than muscle power.[5] This has great significance for labour, for harmony between body and mind, and being able to surrender to the birth process.

It is a good idea to use a chair to help you adopt any vertical head-down positions so that you can unfold gradually, or alternatively slowly walk up a wall with your feet. It is vital to have a good teacher who understands the special needs of pregnancy.

Aerobics must also be specially adapted to pregnancy and a teacher should understand the physiology and stresses of pregnancy. Each exercise session should start with a warm-up, go on to vigorous movement and finish with a cool-down. You can check that your heart is not being made to work too hard by taking your pulse regularly.[6]

In an 'active birth' a woman is free to move around spontaneously as and when she wishes, and is not restrained in any way.[7] In classes beforehand she learns movements and positions which allow maximum opening of her pelvis. If you can find in your area birth classes which incorporate stretching exercises and movements for Active Birth, you have the advantage of combining exercise for pregnancy and rehearsing for labour in which you are upright as much as possible, change position often and give birth squatting, kneeling or on all fours (or in modifications of these positions) rather than reclining or lying down in the 'stranded beetle' position.

Although in the twentieth century the labour bed and delivery table have been treated as essential items of equipment in every hospital, all over the world from time immemorial women have chosen to labour moving around, getting into positions in which they feel most comfortable, and pushing the baby out with their feet planted firmly on the ground and in upright or semi-upright positions. Medieval midwives delivered women on low, horseshoe-shaped birth stools and until the introduction of hospital births it was normal practice for women to walk around during labour and to carry on working in the house or smallholding, often until the onset of the second stage. The postures our great-grandmothers chose were modifications of the squatting, kneeling and crouching postures still used in Third World countries today.[8] In these positions the uterus is not pressing on the largest blood vessel in the lower part of the body, the inferior *vena cava*, so reducing fetal oxygen supply, and gravity helps the delivery of both the baby and the placenta.[9]

A woman in labour tends to be more comfortable upright and walking around, though she may enjoy lying down for short intervals. In a British study by Flynn and Kelly[10] women who were encouraged to move around needed fewer pain-relieving drugs and were sometimes reluctant to get on the bed when they were told they could do so. Their contractions were more effective in opening up the cervix, so the first stage was shorter, and at birth the babies were in better condition than those whose mothers lay in bed.

An upright posture produces greater pressure within the pelvis and lets the uterus form a globular shape during contractions. If you are leaning forward, as a woman usually does spontaneously, the baby's head is tipped forward away from your sacrum – the bone which forms the back of the pelvis. This reduces backache and encourages the rotation of the baby's head into the correct position for delivery.

It is all very well deciding in advance that you would like to be out of bed and walking around during labour, but when it comes to it there often seems to be nowhere else to go and you find yourself wandering around the bed or aimlessly up and down a corridor. It is a good idea to think ahead to some different kinds of movements and positions which you might find comfortable, and which can help you handle pain. These should be practised as early in pregnancy as possible. In the Third World women crouch or squat as a matter of course instead of sitting for all kinds of daily activities. Because in the West we usually sit on chairs it can be uncomfortable to squat or crouch for more than a minute or two; ligaments and muscles in the pelvis and back tend to be stiff and our knees and ankle joints tight. Careful, gentle practice done regularly throughout pregnancy will help you to loosen up progressively for childbirth. Aim for smooth, full, flowing movements and avoid jerky, erratic ones. When a muscle is contracted suddenly or very hard, spasm may result and instead of being flexible and stretched, it springs back and becomes shorter.

Exercises for Active Birth

Many childbirth classes now include both exercises for physical well-being in pregnancy and positions for Active Birth. The concept of Active Birth is based on the idea that the woman in labour is an active birth-giver, not a passive patient. So instead of lying down for doctors and nurses to do things to you, you get into positions which you find comfortable and move around as and when you wish. This means that you are not restricted to a labour bed or even a birth chair but are free to move around on the floor, in a shower, leaning against the wall, the furniture or your birth companion. Changing position as often as you want, you work with the process of birth.

2a A good way to practise squatting.

2b A half-squatting, half-kneeling position which can be very comfortable in labour. Change from left to right knee whenever you want to.

2c   A full kneeling position, leaning forward with support - good for backache.

2d   An all-fours position. Often comfortable with a backache labour.

2e A standing position can feel good if you have someone to lean against.

Exploring different positions

Squatting is most comfortable when you hold on to something firm or someone in front of you, or when you are supported by two helpers, one at each side. When you first start practising squatting, do so for a short time only, and either wear shoes with low heels or slip a pillow under your heels to avoid putting strain on the Achilles tendons. As the muscles stretch you will be able to hold the position for longer and gradually lower your heels to the ground.

Experiment too with *half-squatting, half-kneeling*, with one knee bent down on the floor, the other bent up with your foot on the floor, as this can be even more comfortable in labour than a full squat. Many women spontaneously seek positions in which the pelvis is asymmetric like this, and the tilting of the pelvis, especially if it is combined with pelvic movement, may help the baby's head to rotate into the correct position for delivery.

There are a variety of good *kneeling* positions, too, in which you do not necessarily need to hold on to anything or be supported. Try changing between a position in which you are sitting up on your heels, leaning forward on to a pillow placed on a chair-seat, and further forward still, legs wide apart with your forearms on the floor. A prayer-stool, sold in some shops catering for people with back problems, enables you to kneel with your bottom slightly raised and supported. This could be one of the things you have with you in case you want to use it in labour. Or you may like to kneel with your partner kneeling behind you so that you can have support from his or her thighs. These positions can feel good if you have a backache labour, and they are all ones in which it is easy to give lower back massage or counter-pressure.

Another variation is to get on to *all fours*, knees and arms well apart, so tilting the baby away from the small of your back and forward on to your abdominal wall. This position is excellent for backache, and if the baby's spine lies parallel with yours, with its face and limbs forwards (occipito-posterior position). It can also be comfortable during labour with a baby in the breech position.

Standing is another good position to practise. Explore different ways in which you can use a wall or piece of heavy furniture or lean against your labour companion. Try leaning over a table or on to a window-sill.

With all these positions you do not have to be static. You can change from one to another and then back again. Ask someone to help you – preferably the person who is going to be your birth companion – to experiment with different kinds of movement in each position. See how it feels when you move your pelvis rhythmically. Try rocking, swaying and slow circling. Find ways in which your companion can help you best. Do you want your helper to be still or to move *with* you? Would you like firm holding, massage or light stroking? How can your partner give physical support and also be in a position where you can make eye contact if this is what you want?

Experiment with positions and movements that might be good in the bath or shower. Water can feel wonderfully refreshing in labour.

If you are having your baby in hospital the journey there can be uncomfortable unless you work out in advance easy positions in the car. The back seat is often best. See how pillows can help support your back or can allow you to be on all fours or to recline on your side.

Imagine, too, how you might want to lie if you were feeling extremely tired. On your side is better than on your back. A side-lying position ensures that the heavy uterus is not pressing on vessels through which blood flows back to your heart, so you will not feel dizzy and faint.

Imagine needing to vomit, pass urine or empty your bowels and work out easy positions for these natural functions.

Make a note of the positions and movements you prefer, so that when the time comes there is little chance of getting stuck lying down on your back, or in one position which you dare not change either because your whole body feels too heavy or because you are afraid that the pain will get worse if you do. As pregnancy advances your centre of gravity changes and positions and movements you prefer may change too.

Exercise plans for after the birth

This is the time to make enquiries about exercise or yoga classes after the baby is born. Many classes have crèche facilities so that you can work out knowing that your baby is cared for while you take time to concentrate on your own health. Some cater for mothers and babies together, so that if yours is not sleeping peacefully or enjoying watching, you can include the baby in the movements. A baby a few months' old loves energetic activity and doing exercises together can be great fun.

Even if you cannot get to classes regularly, this is something you can do at home, especially if you have learnt how. One advantage of classes, however, is that you meet other women there, and this social contact helps a lot as you cope with what can be the daunting experience of learning how to be a mother. If you have left your job and are taking time off to get to know your baby, it is important not to become house-bound and socially isolated. For far too many new mothers the high point of the day is a trip to the supermarket. It is hardly surprising that women cut off from all their usual social contacts, who don't see another adult for hours on end, often get depressed. That kind of depression is nothing to do with hormones. It comes from being terribly lonely and not having the emotional and social support you need.

In postnatal exercise classes you and your baby can benefit from the stimulus which comes not only from vigorous activity, but also from having regular outings together and meeting and talking with other women who are going through the same experience.

> In your notebook jot down your plans for exercise after the baby comes, along with addresses and phone numbers which will be useful then.

THE ENVIRONMENT IN PREGNANCY

Whether you are working outside or in the home, or – as with most women – in both places, pregnancy is a time to look at your environment, find out whether it needs improving and, if so, change it if possible.

Are there chemical dangers in the places where you work? Do you breathe clean air? Is the temperature right? (When pregnant you feel hotter.) Can you sit comfortably? Do you have to stand for long periods? Are you in positions in which you get backache, neck-ache, shoulder tension or pain in your legs or feet? Is the lighting good? Are noise levels acceptable?

It is not only the physical environment. It is also a matter of having to deal with the stresses and strains under which you work. Are you under pressure to meet unrealistic deadlines? Are you without any control over your own timetable or unable to plan ahead? Do you work with machines which dictate your pace and allow you too few breathing spaces? Are there enough breaks when you can use the lavatory? (In early and late pregnancy you want to empty your bladder more often than at other times.) Do you feel that you are never able to finish any task properly, that your work has to be skimped because you are pulled in every direction? Are you at too many people's beck and call? Are the hours you work long and exhausting? Are you exposed to sexual harassment at work, having to run the gauntlet of comments about your body, crude jokes or being pawed? If you work outside the home there is the journey to and from work too. Is that stressful?

Living in any big city exposes us all to the stress of constant impersonal and meaningless human contact, the pressure of crowds and of people competing for living space, waiting at the check-out or for the bus, driving in heavy traffic, delayed when we have an urgent appointment – these things irritate, frustrate and exasperate, and they trigger the release of stress hormones which push blood pressure up, increase breathing rates, contract muscles and result in general body tension and mental stress.

Stress is often talked about as if it should not exist. Yet a certain amount of stress is normal – and we can even enjoy it. It is also inevitable. After all, we shall only be completely stress-free when we are dead.

Stress produces challenge, and it is this which can push us out of a rut, make us rethink things we took for granted and stimulate problem-solving and creativity. Stress is there to be *used*.

The ability to enjoy a certain amount of stress depends, however, on important factors in our personal lives and relationships with other people. It is also very difficult to relish stress if we are not basically healthy. When we are physically run down stress can easily tip over into distress.

We are also unlikely to manage stress effectively if we are deprived of any sense of autonomy and personal space because all the time we are at the service of other people, satisfying *their* needs, obeying *their* orders. Stress then results in our feeling put upon and exploited. That is the kind of stress, concerning work both outside the home and inside it, which it is worth acknowledging. We may then negotiate changes with those who are making these demands on us and, if we possibly can, organize life so that stress is reduced.

I realize that, put like this, the list of potential hazards may seem almost endless, your work-place full of threat. This is because most of us have to work under pressure and suffer the effects of living in crowds and in a polluted environment. It is probably impossible to escape this altogether. Sometimes it seems that we are surrounded by dangers that we can do very little about and every time we open a newspaper or watch a TV documentary new hazards are reported. Life in the twentieth century is a dangerous process! And when you are having a baby you become even more alerted to all these risks.

Alarming as they are, it does not follow that there is nothing we can do about them. Even if there are many things we cannot change, there are certainly others that, with determination, effort and by joining with other people who feel the same way, we *can* improve.

This is not just a question of achieving a safe working environment for pregnancy. When poor working conditions affect a pregnant woman's health, or harm an unborn baby, they need improving for the benefit of all of us. Certain pollutants damage sperm too, for example, and a man can become infertile. *All* workers may suffer deterioration in health or, at the very least, not be functioning at full capacity. This is an urgent social issue.

VDUs

If you are working with computers, word processors or video you may be worrying about possible harmful effects on the development of the baby. There has been a good deal of publicity recently about the suspected risks of visual display units – VDUs – for developing babies, especially in the first eight weeks of pregnancy.[1]

The first hazard is that X-rays emitted may be teratogenic (harmful to fetal development). In fact the energy from these X-rays is low and cannot be detected beyond the glass screen of the tube. A study of mothers of babies with birth defects found no evidence that a higher number than usual had worked with VDUs in early pregnancy.[2]

But even if VDUs do not cause birth defects, are women who work with them more likely to have miscarriages? That is the other worry.

The Trades Union Congress recommends that pregnant women should be able to switch to other work because 'worry as a result of uncertainty about VDU work might, itself, prove a significant threat to the success of the pregnancy'.[3]

VDUs certainly adversely affect health in other ways. Furniture and lighting in offices are usually designed for reading and writing at desks and VDUs can be hard on the eyes (though this does not make eyesight deteriorate) and cause a bad working posture. Spots and rashes are sometimes produced on the jaw – a combination of electrostatic fields and a dry atmosphere, coupled with electrostatic charges in synthetic office carpeting, poor ventilation and contaminants in the air. All in all, worry about the possible dangers of VDUs ought to make us re-examine our working conditions generally and improve the environment for everyone.

Pesticides

There has been a lot of publicity about pesticides and their effects on the organs and central nervous system of the developing fetus. If you live and work in the countryside, or just do some gardening – even if that is only with plants in a window-box – you may wonder about the chemicals you are using or to which you may be exposed.

The US Environmental Protection Agency states that approximately a third of the active ingredients of registered pesticides are poisonous and a quarter are highly mutagenic (damage genes) and carcinogenic.[4]

Chlorinated dioxin is known to cause miscarriage, stillbirth and birth defects (cleft palate and kidney abnormalities especially). Dioxin was the active principle of Agent Orange used in Vietnam, and was the chemical sprayed over thousands of people in an explosion at a factory in Seveso, Italy. In Oregon it was used to spray forests and a study by the EPA shows that women had a high rate of miscarriage in that area, most of the babies being lost in June and July, after the peak spraying period in March and April.

When cattle feed on dioxin-sprayed grass, the chemical is concentrated in their fat. Dioxin is also present in the wood preservative pentachlorophenol and in some plant sprays. On the label it may be indicated as 2,4-D, or 2,4,5-T or TCDD (the TC stands for tetrachlorine and the DD for dioxin).

In the USA the Federal Drugs Administration restricts the use of organo-chlorine compounds, including DDT, and organo-phosphates (e.g., malathion) have largely replaced them now. But we do not know if their long-term use is safe. Though they do not cause damage to organs, they may have more subtle effects on the central nervous system and on learning behaviour.

- Before buying or using any pesticide, read the label.
- Check through cupboards where you keep fly sprays and plant pesticides and throw out any which contain toxaphrene or other chlorines.
- If you use organo-phosphates, wear a mask.
- Pyrethrum is probably the safest insecticide for domestic use.
- If any food plants are likely to have been sprayed with a pesticide, wash carefully before cooking or eating raw.
- Always wash your hands after using any pesticide.

Other chemicals

Carbon monoxide in the blood of an unborn baby exceeds that in the mother's blood by up to 15 per cent.[5] It deprives the baby of oxygen and growth may be retarded. Some people living and working in cities have carbon monoxide blood levels of 4 per cent, equal to smoking a pack of cigarettes a day.

If you live in a city and can cut down the time you are exposed to carbon-monoxide-polluted air, it will benefit you and your baby. You may be at greatest risk on the journey to and from work if traffic is heavy at that time. Here are some things you can do:

- Stagger working hours so that you can travel to and from work when there is less build-up of traffic.
- Whenever possible, avoid waiting behind a car with its engine running.
- Avoid jogging where there is heavy traffic; choose a park instead. If the air you have to breathe is contaminated with carbon monoxide, do not run the extra risk of smoking as well, and whenever possible avoid smoky atmospheres.

Three heavy metals, mercury, lead and cadmium, are known to be hazardous, and possibly also nickel and selenium.

Mercury concentration in the brain of the unborn baby is twice that in the mother's brain. In the fifties and sixties mercury poisoning from fish and shellfish affected villages around a bay in southern Japan and babies were born brain-damaged. The source was traced to a plastics factory which discharged its effluent into Minamata Bay. Yet even when this was known, a further outbreak occurred in another part of Japan resulting from similar industrial discharge. Mercury is also used as a fungicide. There was a disaster in Iraq caused by grain which had been treated with methyl mercury bought from Mexico. Though there was a warning on the sack that it should not be used for making bread, this warning was in Spanish.

Lead poisoning results in damage to sperm and miscarriage. Evidence as to whether it causes birth defects is conflicting. But when young women workers at a chemical factory at Willow Island, West Virginia, wanted to keep jobs which required exposure to lead dust they had to agree to be sterilized. Five women were sterilized and some later regretted it.[6]

Yet a woman is not just a container for a fetus or a set of ova. Her own health is important, and if that is damaged by exposure to lead she should not have to work with it. And since lead poisoning not only harms sperm but can adversely affect men's health too, men should not be forced to suffer exposure to lead in their work either. As a speaker at a Women's TUC conference said: 'While women are being discriminated against, men are being conned.'

The women workers at Willow Island sued the company, Cyanamid. As a result of this political action and the publicity it generated, maximum lead levels have been fixed by law for all US workers.

Cadmium is used in electro-plating factories, from where it is discharged into the sewage system, is a constituent of tobacco smoke, and is produced as rubber tyres wear out. In high concentrations it too can cause birth defects and growth retardation.

Another dangerous chemical, ethylene oxide, is used by nurses to sterilize instruments, and if they are in early pregnancy can cause miscarriage. Other people who may come into contact with ethylene oxide are workers in the pharmaceutical industry who sterilize drugs, and others employed in factories where certain kinds of food are chemically sterilized. Glutaraldehyde and formaldehyde are safer chemical agents than ethylene oxide.[7]

Hexachlorophene, a cleansing agent much used in hospitals, aniline, benzene and turpentine may also cause birth defects. Occasional contact with these substances is unlikely to be dangerous, but if a pregnant woman works with them daily she and her baby are exposed to special risk.

Women are often exposed indirectly to dangers which their partners encounter in *their* work-places. If your partner, or anyone else in the family, does work which involves contamination with chemical or metal dust, work clothes should either be laundered at the place of work or be put in a plastic bag before they are brought into the home and then tipped straight into the washing machine. Dust can also be carried in hair, even when protective clothing is worn. Workers should shower and wash their hair to avoid bringing this dust into the home.

The dangers of asbestos are now well known. Inhaled asbestos can cause a rare form of cancer. Research has focused on disease caused by working with asbestos (in shipyards or car factories, for example) rather than on possible effects on the unborn baby, but animal studies show that asbestos dust can pass through the placenta. So avoid contact with flaking asbestos – on an old ironing board, for example, or a deteriorating insulation panel behind an electric heater – for both your own and the baby's sake.

When jobs are few, women may be sacked on the grounds that they are unsuitable because they may get pregnant and the work could cause miscarriage, premature birth, stillbirth or birth handicaps. They lose their jobs and the place is still not cleaned up. The fetus is protected at the expense of the woman, and – since chemical pollution, for example, can harm male fertility at levels as low as those set for women – at the expense of male workers too. The woman is treated merely as a potential container for a baby. The man is ignored, considered too tough to be affected, and forced to go on being exposed to these toxins.

Pollution at work is not a matter for women only. It is a challenge for all of us.

Buildings

Cavity foam insulation is used in many modern office blocks, public buildings, hospitals, schools and homes. Formaldehyde is sprayed into the wall cavities and produces a toxic gas as it dries. This usually disperses into the air outside, but if it leaks into the building it can cause headaches, breathlessness, a runny nose, eye irritation, coughs and colds, skin rashes, sore throats, drowsiness and lapses of memory. Sometimes this gas is still present in the air long after the building has been insulated, and its presence can be detected by a strong chemical smell. There is no evidence that this could affect the fetus, but anything which makes you that uncomfortable is in any case best avoided.

Old buildings sometimes have lead water pipes. You are more likely to find them in your home than in a modern office block or factory. They contaminate drinking water, especially if it is naturally soft or if a softener is used, since soft water dissolves lead. The placenta is unable to filter out lead, which passes through and becomes concentrated on the side of the placenta nearest the baby. It can cause genetic damage.

You can tell if pipes are made of lead because they are dark and rather soft – a knife cuts through them rather than just leaving a scratch. They should be replaced with copper. If you cannot avoid drinking water from lead pipes, let it run for 30 seconds to clear any deposits. First thing in the morning, allow water to run for a couple of minutes to flush out any lead deposits which have built up overnight.

Action for a healthier work-place

Either on your own, or better still with a group of women colleagues at work, and your trade union Health and Safety Representative if you have one, or with other women who also work at home, critically examine your work-place to see if it provides a healthy environment and how it could be improved. Make your own checklist for this. If it is difficult to find out whether, for example, the air is polluted in any way, devise a plan of action to get information about this. You may need to get advice from an environmental health officer (contact your local council) or the Health and Safety Executive. Trade unions can also help. Make a note of all the things which concern you. Seek a single standard to control each hazard at work to ensure maximum protection for all workers, male and female.

Food habits are also likely to be affected by your work. Whether you eat in the staff restaurant, grab a snack wherever and whenever you can because of pressure of work, or entertain a lot as part of your work, look at Chapter 4. It may suggest improvements you could make in nutrition.

If there are no smoking-free zones in your place of work and you have to breathe tobacco smoke, this is another issue you may want to consider, bearing in mind the material on smoking and pregnancy in Chapter 3.

If air is polluted use a fan or air filter, or improve ventilation by opening a window when possible.

Use a mask or other protective clothing if necessary.

If you decide that stress is a major problem at work, consider action you could take which would reduce it. It is not a trivial matter. Constant excessive stress can make people physically and mentally ill. Many medical conditions – asthma, migraine and other headaches, eczema, indigestion, constipation, high blood pressure and heart problems are stress-related. Here are some of the questions you may want to ask yourself and discuss with other women who do similar work:

- Do you need to be more assertive?
- Can you organize regular breaks from work, especially if it is monotonous or especially demanding?
- Can your work be rearranged so that particularly stressful tasks do not follow immediately one on the other and you have a 'breather' in between them?
- Do you need more time on your own, or, alternatively, working alongside other people?
- Can the job be done in a different sequence or methods employed which would make it less stressful?
- Can noise be reduced and lighting be improved?
- Can you cut down the number of interruptions which make it difficult to concentrate?

There may be other things which can help too:

- Taking time for relaxation and learning how to relax physically and mentally.

- Getting more exercise.
- Being out of doors sometimes rather than in a building all day.
- Sharing the work or getting someone else to take over part of it.
- And, perhaps, also reducing the demands you make on yourself.

These may all be ways for you to manage stress more effectively.

If you are worried

What if you have already been exposed to chemicals or enormous stress which you feel might have harmed you or the baby? Since the greatest effect is in the first eight weeks of pregnancy, even before you knew you were pregnant, what should you be doing? What *can* you do?

Take comfort that the chances are high that your baby will be perfect. Our concern about teratogens in the environment has come about through large-scale statistical studies involving enormous numbers of births. Even with powerful chemicals, the chances of your baby being harmed are very low indeed.

If you are healthy, well nourished and do not smoke, any effects of poisons on your unborn child are much reduced. If damage had been done in those first eight weeks the chances are that you would have had a miscarriage. A great many miscarriages occur because there is something wrong with the developing embryo.

One consequence of raised consciousness about pregnancy and our rights as women is that we develop an often frightening sense of responsibility and have to learn how to handle the anxiety that stems from this. Anxiety can be used constructively if it leads to linking up with others in order to improve the conditions under which we work.

7

EMOTIONAL CHANGES

In one sense, of course, a woman has no choice about the emotions she feels during pregnancy. They just come and have to be lived with, the good and the bad. In another sense, you *do* have choice. You can acknowledge your feelings or try to escape from them by denying them. You can seek to understand why you are feeling this way or you can dismiss that as too disturbing or dangerous, or avoid acknowledging your emotions because you think it is wrong or silly to have them. You can decide to be open about how you feel with someone close to you – your partner or a friend – or you can put on an act of being placid and unruffled throughout pregnancy.

All this doesn't just apply to emotions like fear and anxiety about whether the baby will be normal. It is sometimes a temptation to suppress or try to hide from others feelings of tremendous elation, even ecstasy, because they seem 'silly' too, and 'no one would understand'.

In the following pages I want to look at some of the dominant emotional states of pregnancy so that you can explore how you feel, understand what you share with other women and decide if there is any action you can take in response to these emotional challenges.

Pregnancy is for some women a time of deep emotional satisfaction and an oasis of content. There is a feeling of being in tune with life. Senses are heightened. For one woman the first crisp, cold air of winter produces a tingle of excitement. When storms toss the trees and she is heavy with child she sometimes feels as if she, too, is like a great tree, its roots deep in the earth. For another, pregnant in the springtime, flower shoots pushing through the earth and fronds of green unfurling on the branches echo the physical sense of life moving inside her body. As a woman lies in the sun, her abdomen like a great curved melon soaking up its heat, she may feel a tremendous inner energy, the power of her uterus, now cradling her baby, which will later be strong to knead and squeeze the child out of her body. Watching the sea, she senses the movement of waves and the rush and swirl of water as if it flows, too, in the inner world of her uterus. There is a symmetry with nature, a unity with the elements, which brings a feeling of rightness about her body.

We do not often talk about these feelings because they are so distinctly womanly that it can be difficult to find words to describe them. They are not in the male language we normally have to use. So we tend to be embarrassed talking about them, or even never grasp the experience for ourselves – because there are no words with which to understand and encapsulate it.

Even a woman for whom pregnancy was an accident, or who conceived before she was quite ready for it, may go through it with delight. And though weary with the heavy load she carries, there are still likely to be precious times when she feels her whole body glowing and radiant with life.

Yet an inescapable fact about pregnancy is that – emotionally – each woman is as if on the rim of the void. More than any explorer in frozen wastes of ice, more than any sailor in an expanse of uncharted ocean, she is alone in the face of a momentous event, the drama of birth, which is going to open her body and bring from its depths a new human being. She has only to think about that to feel awe at the magnitude of what must happen, to know eager anticipation and wonder – and sometimes also fear.

The paramount and overwhelming theme of every pregnancy is that of change. Nothing stays as it was. Everything is in a state of flux. The woman's appearance changes from one month to the next. Emotions change, even perhaps from day to day. Pregnancy is growth. It is also metamorphosis – for the child from embryo to fetus and from fetus to newborn baby. For the woman it brings a gradual and inexorable swelling and ripening until her body is ready for birth. In terms of emotions and relationships, it transforms her into a different kind of social being, with often incredibly passionate bonds of love and responsibility to one small human creature, as she becomes a mother.

This nine months' journey may be marked by some of the most profound and powerful emotions a human being can ever feel. It is often claimed that pregnant women are placid and, indeed, many women are concerned that they may get cow-like, their brains so softened by maternity that they are incapable of logical thought. The recurrent advertising stereotype of pregnancy is that of an expectant mother knitting contentedly in the lamplight or dreamily picking daisies in a meadow, far removed from and untouched by the turmoil of everyday life. An expectant mother, these advertisements seem to be saying, is fulfilled as she dreams of the coming baby. A vessel for the new life, her mind is tranquil, and no needs of her own intrude on this harmony.

The reality is different. Pregnancy is often a time of deeply disturbing emotional conflicts and many women are exposed to stresses from outside – in the environment and in their relationships – which make of it an arduous passage. Far from being insulated from the external world and its stresses, it may all have a greater and more painful impact, as the woman faces the life crisis of birth.

The first emotional conflicts may come when she realizes that she has conceived. However much a baby is wanted, however careful the planning, the reality of discovering that you are pregnant can be almost unbelievable, thrilling and strangely disquieting. For now you have to face up to it. You have started something which cannot be stopped except by a deliberate act of termination or an accident of nature. There is an inevitability about the whole process which can be both awe-inspiring and alarming.

The first movements are felt between 18 and 20 weeks and from that moment you are constantly reminded that there is someone else inside you. This creature is not just part of your body, but has its own life and, though still growing from and dependent on yours, is nevertheless distinct and different. Sometimes it feels wonderful to have this other life developing inside you. At others it may feel like an intrusion and you think of the fetus merely as a kind of parasite – and then, perhaps, feel a wave of guilt at having such thoughts. This sense of two people in one body can be threatening. Even a woman who welcomes her pregnancy is likely to have times when she asks herself, 'Is this what I really want?' There is nothing abnormal about these feelings. There are times in almost any pregnancy when a woman feels that her body is completely taken over and that she has been swallowed up and has disappeared inside it. She may wonder whether she will ever be able to find herself again.

Sally felt like that through much of her pregnancy. She had been an athlete and a keen horsewoman, but after she had some bleeding in early pregnancy, even though there was no evidence that her riding had caused it, her doctor advised her not to ride again until after the baby was born. She said:

> I hated being pregnant. I hated looking pregnant. I had always been slim and taken pride in my body. I thought my swollen body was revolting. And mentally I felt that I was losing my grip. The doctor treated me like an irresponsible child.

For some women pregnancy entails a loss of identity, a death of self. They resist what is happening to their bodies and try to carry on exactly as before. It can be a very frightening experience. Becoming a patient, and being forced to surrender one's identity as an adult capable of making rational judgements, increases this sense of loss of self. One way of counteracting it is to get together with other pregnant women to start exploring childbirth choices and weighing up the alternatives, and thus start functioning as an adult again. A woman who feels that she is trapped inside her pregnant body may feel quite different once she starts exercise classes and learns how to breathe and relax and prepare for Active Birth, since the movements learnt in groups like these help her towards greater harmony with her body.

Any link between such emotions and how a woman feels about her baby once it is born is extremely tenuous. It is astonishing how often one who hated pregnancy falls head-over-heels in love with her baby at birth or in the days following. For some women there is a vast difference between the feeling of having a baby inside the uterus and a baby in their arms and they can welcome one, but not the other. (For there are women, too, who like being pregnant but feel emotionally numb for a time once the baby puts in an appearance.)

Many women say they respond with strong emotions to suffering, whether of human beings or animals. Tears come quickly, and television programmes which extol violence or vividly depict the consequences of war, and press photographs of starving children with their swollen bellies and stick-like limbs, prove unbearably distressing. It is as if approaching motherhood sensitizes you to the needs not only of your own child, but of all the world's children. This increased awareness of suffering, the overwhelming compassion and urge to help those hungry and in need, is an important part of the spontaneous emotional changes which precede birth. They prepare us to nurture a child. The world is in short supply of these qualities of nurturing. We often clamp down on such emotions because the exposed nerve causes too much pain. Yet this nurturing concern which spills over from pregnancy and the experience of motherhood should not be dismissed lightly. It is important in politics – in the peace movement, for example – in bringing aid to famine-stricken people, and in the struggle for social and economic justice. It can be a power for good in the world, and, difficult as it can be to do so, perhaps this new emotional vulnerability should be welcomed.

A major doubt in a woman's mind may be whether she is ready to be a mother. If you have never had much to do with babies or thought of yourself as a mother you may wonder whether you have any 'maternal instincts'. In human beings mothering is learned behaviour. Though there is an instinctual element, no one could rely on instincts alone to see her through the highly complex series of tasks involved in being a mother in today's society. We learn from books, the media and parent classes. But we probably learn most by simply watching other women with their babies – seeing how they handle and respond to them, what they do, how they talk to, hold, rock and soothe them – and pick up information often when we are least aware of it. It is very different from academic learning.

Many women who have never had the chance of caring for a small child and who do not have younger brothers and sisters lack confidence in their mothering skills. But you will find that your baby soon teaches you what to do and will leave you in no doubt about what she likes, when she needs to be fed, played with and talked to, and exactly what makes her feel comfortable and contented. You do not have to rely on 'maternal instincts' for that.

One element in worry about what happens *after* the baby comes is concern about the sheer practicalities of looking after a baby. If you are going back to your job immediately, or after an interval, getting good childcare may be looming large in your mind: its cost, whether it is going to be reliable, and what you can do if it does not work out. It pays not only to plan ahead but to make all your contacts, with alternative arrangements if your first choice does not come to anything, as early in pregnancy as you possibly can. Otherwise you may spend the whole nine months worrying about it.

You may not yet have decided about going back to your job. It is best to keep options open if you can, anyway, since no matter how sure you may be now, you may feel differently once the baby is born. A woman who plans to go back to work immediately often feels she cannot leave her baby, and one who plans on being a full-time mother finds that it is driving her up the wall! So all plans should be flexible.

Whether or not she is working outside the home, every woman with children needs a good informal support network of people who can help out, or substitute for her, when the going gets tough. In the days of large extended families this existed automatically, but many modern women are alone and isolated. You might think any woman ought to be able to cope with one child at least, but a first-time mother with a new baby needs people to help her feel that what she is doing is right and that, even though she is a complete novice, she is a 'good enough' mother. It is not so much advice she needs as someone to listen and to take over tasks such as shopping, cooking and cleaning.

Many women having their first child are far from their own families and friends with whom they grew up. They are preoccupied with their jobs, and social contacts have been mostly with work colleagues, many of whom may not have children. They may never have met the people living in the same street. If they move before the baby is born, or soon afterwards, as many do, they know no one at all in the area. At the stage when a woman is completely preoccupied with the baby and finds that the day-to-day tasks of baby-care take up all her time, it can be very difficult to make new friends.

So it is important to make plans well before the baby is born to develop survival strategies for afterwards. Anxiety now can provide the spur for planning ahead like this. You can build up a support network both by having a list of emergency contacts whom you can pay to take over essential tasks (your phone book may be able to help here) and also by setting out to meet people, through clubs and voluntary associations – childbirth, church and women's groups, for instance – with whom you can create a mutual support network. There is a list of organizations, many of which are also pressure groups for change, on pp. 311–15.

Besides a peer support group of women roughly the same age and all coping with the same kinds of challenges in their lives, it is helpful to have older women friends who are not trying to cope at present with the same day-to-day problems. They may not do things quite your way but can still be a valuable resource, and their experience and confidence stands you in good stead when you are feeling overwhelmed. It is fashionable nowadays to deride and criticize the help that such older women can give. It can be a way in which some professionals try to isolate new mothers from the support they can get from other women, preferring that they should rely on *their* advice alone. But it is not really advice that you will need. It is someone to listen, the warmth of friendship, someone who can give you an occasional break from the baby and allow you to rediscover a little personal space.

When Maureen and Jim had their baby they got to know a woman in her sixties who lived a few doors up and whose husband had died recently. She was obviously lonely and her own grandchildren were half a continent away. Mrs Smith was worried about insurance and other money matters with which she had to deal – something she had never done before. Maureen and Jim were able to help with these and Mrs Smith, in her turn, was delighted to do baby-sitting and became an adopted grandmother.

Many support networks grow spontaneously, but when you are pregnant it is risky to leave your post-baby network to chance, and to do so causes unnecessary anxiety. So reach out and make friends now!

Loves playing with the baby. 'Sings to her, but 10 minutes is enough

Husband. Super cook and washer-up. Takes over completely when I need rest

Me with my support plan

My mother does all the things that I hate doing. I daren't argue about it

The little person this is all about

Fellow parents who live next door. We have their 2-year-old to stay if they go out, and ours loves to stay with them at night

Teenager. Takes the baby for a walk after school in good weather. Amuses her at home in early evening while I concentrate on the toddler

More parents. Live in next street. Baby of same age

Her son. Runs errands, takes messages, plays with the baby

Another parent. We swap things; baby-sit for each other

Health Visitor

Family doctor

Occasional cleaning lady, baby minder. Straightforward because I pay her

One woman's support group.

Some pregnant women are tortured with fear that the baby may be abnormal, and even those who dismiss such thoughts from their minds during the day-time often feel anxious at night. Mental handicap is the thing they most dread. One woman said:

> I lie there thinking that I could face almost any physical handicap but I just don't have the courage to deal with a mentally handicapped child. Last night was awful. Yesterday I saw a woman leading a Down's syndrome girl by the hand. Her tongue was hanging out. She must have been in her twenties. I thought, 'What if my baby grows up like that?' I couldn't face it! It would wreck our lives!

It is not difficult for any pregnant woman to think back to something that occurred in the first weeks of pregnancy which might have harmed her baby: drugs, alcohol, cigarette smoke or something else which could have interrupted fetal development. Few of us live in such an unpolluted environment that we can't point to some toxic chemical which might have caused damage. As one woman said:

> I worry about a lot of things because, however careful I am, I can't be sure that the baby isn't being exposed to poisonous chemicals. At the weekend we went hiking. It was great to get out of the city. But farmers were spraying the crops – I don't know what with. The air was quite still at first, but after we had been walking for about an hour a wind got up and I got really scared. We turned back. It spoilt the day and last night I had a terrible nightmare about a deformed baby.

Occasionally a woman who suffers from anxiety is prescribed drugs which add further to her fear that the baby will be abnormal. Heather, for example, had been taking tranquillizers over a period of nine years. 'Though I reduced my dosage by half before becoming pregnant, I took tranquillizers through my pregnancy,' she said. 'I was very, very scared about the effect of the drugs on the baby. I couldn't believe the irresponsibility of what I had done and felt my baby and I would be blighted for life.' She needed to talk this through with her doctor. But unfortunately she felt so guilty about taking the tranquillizers that she never dared raise the subject with her. If you have medicines for any chronic condition it is wise to have a discussion about this with your doctor well *before* you get pregnant. You can then decide whether to reduce them, cut them out or switch to another kind, or whether, if the effects of the illness would be worse than any side-effects of the drugs, it would be more sensible to go on taking them.

Stress in a job may also cause anxiety during pregnancy. Catherine, for example, was a psychiatric nurse working with patients who were physically as well as mentally sick:

> Most could do very little for themselves. There was a lot of lifting and bathing, as well as the occasional aggressive and violent outburst. I was terribly afraid that the baby would be hurt in some way.

She had to keep on working because they needed the money. But it might have been possible for her to be moved to less demanding work in the hospital. Her anxiety was obviously rooted in reality and it certainly could not be dismissed as merely a figment of a pregnant woman's imagination due to special emotional vulnerability.

It is well known that German measles (rubella) in the first eight weeks of pregnancy can damage the fetal heart, brain, sight and hearing. Diana had not been immunized against rubella and contracted the disease shortly after she became pregnant:

> I went for a blood test. It came back positive. My husband and I were absolutely devastated. We desperately wanted a baby. We told the doctor that we would continue the pregnancy. We were told that there was a 20 per cent chance of the baby being born with a handicap of the eyes or ears. From that day on till the end of my pregnancy we went through hell. Some days we could discuss it. Other days we refused to accept that anything could be wrong. I was under terrible strain. Not many days went by without crying either in the bathroom at work or at night in bed. I will never know how my husband and I survived those everlasting 40 weeks. [Her baby was perfect.]

A woman who has lost a baby previously from a late miscarriage or stillbirth is often waiting for the same thing to happen with this pregnancy. She may be on her guard until the time has passed when she miscarried before, or right until the baby is safely delivered. An experience like that casts its shadow forward, and even though you feel you have come through the grief and are now starting out with fresh hope, it is there in the background and may haunt the present pregnancy. There may be special dates in pregnancy when you think, 'At this stage last time I felt very much as I do now. Perhaps this means that something is wrong,' or something else happens which is like an echo of the previous pregnancy and so gives rise to anxiety.

Janice had a stillborn baby two years ago. She rang me after a visit to her doctor:

He said, 'You leave the worrying to me. That's what I'm here for.' He obviously forgot, but he said that before when I told him I couldn't feel much kicking in my last pregnancy.

When a pregnancy has started soon after the death of another child, without enough time to grieve over the loss, a mother may also feel guilty about replacing the dead baby. A woman who had a cot death was advised by her doctor to get pregnant again as soon as possible, and conceived a few months after the baby's death. She told me:

> We bought a lot of things when I was pregnant with Roseann [the baby who died]. I can't help feeling it's all wrong to use them for this baby. It's like closing the door on her – as if I don't care any more.

Another woman, who had a stillbirth, said:

> I keep thinking, 'The baby would have been a year old now,' and wondering if this baby will look like her. Sometimes it is almost as if she has come back and I'm still pregnant with *her*. It's as if I want to make amends to her, give her the chance of life she lost.

Grieving takes many months. Some women need a year or more. A pregnancy which begins before the mourning process is completed may result in very mixed and disturbing feelings.

Often when things have gone wrong and a baby has died, parents have found it very difficult to get full and accurate information about why it happened. Sometimes doctors themselves don't know. But many parents feel that the true facts are being withheld from them by doctors in case of litigation. This may be true.

With the next pregnancy a woman usually feels an urgent need to *know* and be quite sure that nothing is being hidden from her. The best thing is to make this absolutely clear to your doctor. Anne's last pregnancy ended in the stillbirth of a baby with multiple handicaps. When she was pregnant again she asked her obstetrician to give her full and frank information:

> He encouraged me to listen to the fetal heart and when I had an ultrasound scan took time to show both of us our baby's limbs, the heart beating and all the internal organs. We could see the fully formed spine and even watched the bladder emptying. And he described exactly how he was going to measure the baby's growth and development and reassured me that all was well.

A previous abortion, which a woman thinks she has put behind her – even one a long time back – can cause feelings of inexplicable depression and anxiety in the next pregnancy.

Beth was talking to me about her overwhelming fear that her baby would be malformed. She did not go through a day without brooding on this. It was only when we talked about the termination she had three years ago, and her feelings then, that she said: 'I feel that this baby is going to be abnormal as a punishment for getting rid of that baby.'

However rational we want to be, many of us have a similar dread of retribution during a pregnancy following a previous abortion. It isn't just a matter of having lost a baby before, but of abortion. Women who had a previous miscarriage are not especially likely to feel like this.[1]

Pregnancy may be marred by dread of going into hospital and what 'they' will do to you. This is another realistic anxiety about loss of autonomy.

Robin, for example, spent six months trying to find an obstetrician who was willing to help her have a natural birth. The first 'treated me like a schoolgirl, in a very condescending way', and it was not until 26 weeks that she was able to switch to a doctor who had newly arrived in the area and was interested in natural birth. He worked with her to build a personal birth plan. Only after this was she able to relax and start to enjoy her pregnancy.

Anxiety which stems from being powerless and having other people make all the decisions about you and your baby can be dispelled only by constructive action. It entails either improving communication and understanding with your care-givers and shifting the balance of power, or changing them and the environment in which you give birth. There is no easy solution by means of facile reassurance, breathing deeply or meditation. You should not have to try and change yourself to fit the system. Somehow you have to change the system to suit your needs.

It can take a long time to get over a distressing labour and look forward with joy to the next one. People sometimes advise you to try and 'forget', but that is impossible. A better way is to find out all you can about exactly what went wrong last time, and why, so that you can make sense of what happened and prepare for the coming birth with fresh knowledge and understanding.

Elaine's previous labour was a ghastly experience. She had gone into it relying on the obstetrician to do everything for the best, because he was the expert. It turned out to be a high-tech labour culminating in a forceps delivery. She said that one of the worst things about it was that a crowd of medical students piled into the room to watch the delivery and the obstetrician talked to them rather than to her: 'I was merely Exhibit A. It was,' she added, 'like a gang rape.' With this pregnancy she changed her obsterician and made sure such a thing could never happen again:

> I wrote a list of questions before I went to see my obstetrician and had a long talk with my husband, so that he understood exactly what I wanted. He agreed to come with me to talk with the doctor and was as concerned as I was to make sure that I could have this baby the way *I* wanted. I stressed that, even if intervention was necessary, I would like an intimate atmosphere.

Fear of birth itself is very complex. It is often a mixture of anxiety about being deprived of autonomy, trapped in a situation completely outside your control, being exposed as inadequate and worthless, and fear that you will not be able to handle pain. Worry that the baby will be malformed or that it will die – or that it will be dreadfully malformed and will *not* die – and fear of injury to yourself, even fear that *you* might die, are all part of this pervading anxiety that many women experience, often in the dead of night.

It is important to be able to talk about birth fears openly with someone who understands and does not dismiss them. Your childbirth teacher might be the right person, or a sympathetic doctor or midwife. In childbirth classes where there is full and free discussion, women are often surprised to discover that others share the same fears and many find this sharing very helpful.

For most women anxiety in pregnancy is concentrated on the birth, which is perceived as a time of testing, and even, by some, as one of judgement and punishment. The dread of pain is only one aspect of this, which is why a doctor's reassurance that pain-relieving drugs are readily available and there is no need for any woman to suffer in labour is largely irrelevant.

One way of dealing with fear of birth is to take constructive action so that you feel well prepared to cope with whatever challenges it presents. That means understanding exactly what happens and what labour feels like in its different phases, and knowing what you can do to help yourself. Those looming fears can be replaced with confident action to work *with* your body instead of against it and, regardless of whether it turns out that you can do it all by yourself, or require help to get the baby born, to approach birth as an active and creative experience.

In any major transitional phase of life there is bound to be anxiety, even if we do not always acknowledge it. It has an important function in stimulating us to seek information, make changes and adapt to new tasks. Anxiety can be used and worked with.

Spend a little time to think of your own anxieties. Cast your mind back to the beginning of pregnancy and make a note of anything that worried you when you first realized you were pregnant. The worries you started out with may have disappeared. If so, think how this happened and make a note of what occurred. You may, for example, have made personal contact with a care-giver who was previously just a shadowy and rather ominous figure. You may have got hold of important information you needed. You may have someone who can give you emotional support and understanding, or be in a group of pregnant women or couples who are helping each other.

Now look at any anxieties that are still on your mind and see what you can do to use them constructively and so reduce their power. The first step is often to talk about them with someone who can accept that you feel like this.

It isn't always realized that fathers can be very anxious but, because they are not pregnant themselves, feel that they should not express their worries. Whoever is going to be your support person in labour, whether or not it is your partner, may be apprehensive about what is going to happen, too. Talking together about this gives an opportunity for your relationship to grow and for each of you to show what you need from the other.

Sex

In the first few months of pregnancy you may find that you go off sex, or prefer gentle stroking and affectionate cuddling to sexual intercourse. Many women feel tenderness and subtlety is lacking in their relationship with a sexual partner, whether or not they are pregnant, and in pregnancy this feeling that sex should be slower, gentler and more caring often crystallizes with still more clarity. You may want to take the opportunity to discuss this with your partner so that pregnancy can draw you closer together rather than driving you apart, as it does some couples.

There is nothing like nausea and vomiting to turn your thoughts from sex and make you feel drained of energy and very negative about your body. Fear of miscarriage also puts a damper on sex, and both partners may be very frightened of somehow dislodging the developing embryo. For many women, too, the medicalizing of pregnancy results in a feeling that their bodies are no longer their own and that they are primarily patients. One element in this is loss of the normal control we have over our bodies and having to hand over responsibility for them to professional care-givers.

Nausea and vomiting, and the tiredness which is common at the beginning of pregnancy, do not usually last longer than three months, and then you may suddenly feel completely different. As one woman told me: 'After the morning sickness was over I felt like a queen!' For a woman, feeling good about yourself like that, rather than stimulation of the genital organs, is the basis for enjoying sex.

In the middle months you may feel more quickly aroused than usual and enjoy sex a lot. This is partly because of the excitement of knowing that the baby is growing inside you, partly because you and your partner share happiness in the pregnancy, and often feel really clever – as if this were the first baby ever to be conceived – and partly because pressure of enlarged blood vessels in your pelvis and against your pelvic floor muscles and vagina has a physically arousing effect. As the pregnancy becomes obvious, women often say they like their bodies more, feel more 'mature', 'womanly', 'feminine', 'fulfilled', 'proud', 'special' and 'wonderful'. 'I loved to be big,' Lindsey said. 'I felt very attractive. Love-making was better than before and I had more powerful orgasms.'

In her fifth month of pregnancy, Angela is in a state of almost continuous arousal:

> My body is now at its most attractive. My hair is soft and sleek, my skin taut and smooth, my cheeks softly glowing. I'm very aware and proud of my firm, rounded breasts and belly. My nipples are erect and big with dark areolas. I masturbate to orgasm at least twice a day. I am enjoying sex to the full in the knowledge that I may only have another four or five weeks of such fun before our sex life becomes curtailed because I feel too cumbersome.

For some women this sexual exhilaration continues right through pregnancy. Sara told me that she enjoyed sex so much she began to worry that she was abnormal and asked the doctor if there was something wrong with her:

He said I was one of the lucky ones. I enjoyed it up until the night I had the baby. We made love at twelve-thirty and my waters broke at three while I was asleep. I kept thinking they would know in hospital, but no one said or asked anything.

She felt rather bewildered because her increased sexual drive did not fit with her image of maternity. Our culture creates an antithesis between sexuality on the one hand and motherhood on the other, as if pregnancy and birth were at the polar extreme to the passion which originally created them. Women are now re-discovering the sexuality of pregnancy and birth.

Even so, as the baby grows and she gets larger a woman is unlikely to enjoy intercourse if her partner is rough, insensitive to her needs or too quick, and many women say they get pleasure from masturbation in pregnancy – sometimes for the first time. 'I was surprised by my increased drive to masturbate,' one woman said. 'It didn't fit the maternal image at all but I masturbated regularly to orgasm, though I couldn't have orgasms with my husband.' It may be that her husband could have learnt something from her about where and how to caress her. Pregnancy can sometimes throw up difficulties like this in a sexual relationship, but can also provide an opportunity to explore sexual feelings more deeply.

Many women find the last weeks difficult because they are too tired to enjoy sex and feel heavy and distended. Some have a very negative picture of their bodies. 'I felt like a whale,' one woman told me. And another: 'My stretch marks look like a map of the world. I feel very ugly. I have not wanted to make love as I have a lot of heartburn and am extremely uncomfortable, and I can't wait to get some sort of figure back!' If this is how you feel, a loving partner can give reassurance by reaffirming delight in your body and helping you feel good about it.

Some men are anxious about sex in pregnancy and very frightened of hurting the woman or the baby, and as a result they withdraw from the physical contact she may be longing for desperately. Even though it may seem to you unfeminine and 'demanding' to ask for it outright, it is important to bring this into the open and say what you want. Otherwise you each retreat into a private shell.

It often happens, too, that just as a woman is feeling sexually exuberant in mid-pregnancy she discovers that her partner seems to have switched off. This can occur because of fear of harming the pregnancy or, sometimes, dislike of the pregnant body and its curves and fullness. Men do not often care to admit that they are afraid, and try to maintain a casual nonchalance which women may interpret as withdrawal of love. 'I thought my husband found me repulsive,' one woman told me, 'as he abstained totally from sex during my pregnancy. However, after much talking and agonizing he told me it was not revulsion at my body, but his fear of hurting the unborn child.' It is sad that it was not until after the baby was born that this couple got down to talking about it.

A man may also treat a pregnant woman as 'not sexy, but sacred', in another woman's words, and deliberately squash all erotic feeling because he believes it is inappropriate or wrong. Some women feel like this too: 'My body felt sacred and special. Love-making ceased as soon as the pregnancy was confirmed.'

Right at the end of pregnancy a man who was fairly carefree about sex earlier on may be almost overwhelmed by a sense of responsibility for this new life and fear that he may hurt the woman:

> In the last three months my husband became increasingly reluctant to have intercourse. He still wanted to be touched, kissed and caressed and wanted me to stimulate him to orgasm, but he wouldn't touch me. At the time I thought he didn't fancy me. Now that we've talked about it I realize that he was just scared of hurting me.

Not all men are like this, of course. Sometimes a woman who does not feel erotic in any way has a partner who is really turned on by pregnancy. Jo did not enjoy her pregnant body at all, and could not understand how her partner could: 'But he said I was daft. He couldn't have wanted me more and he thought I was beautiful when pregnant.'

An American study suggested that intercourse in late pregnancy causes premature rupture of the membranes and resulting infection. But the same researchers then discovered that the infection was the cause of the membrane rupture, not the consequence, and that there was no relation between premature rupture and the number of times a couple said they had intercourse. However, if an amniotic fluid infection is present, sexual intercourse is likely to make it more severe.[2] This means that if a pregnancy is going well and you are feeling healthy, you can trust your own feelings to do what is right for you and make love as often as you want. But it also means that if there is premature leaking of amniotic fluid, even though slight, or you are feeling run down and ill yourself, it would be sensible not to have intercourse and to find other ways of showing your love for each other instead.

Semen is rich in prostaglandins which ripen and soften the cervix at the end of pregnancy. When you explore an unripe cervix with your finger, it feels like the hard tip of your nose. A ripe cervix feels like a soft, relaxed mouth. One way of inducing labour is to introduce prostaglandin gel into the cervix to prepare it for labour, and if the baby is ready to be born this will actually start contractions, often after some hours.

If you notice any bleeding after intercourse and are not yet within three weeks of your due date, it may be wiser, therefore, to avoid intercourse and enjoy 'pleasuring', stroking and cuddling instead. If you are near term or past the date when your baby is due, intercourse is not only harmless but may help labour start, especially if combined with nipple stimulation. Lie still for half an hour after intercourse, while your partner continues to suck and stroke your breasts. It is one of the pleasantest ways there is to start labour, and even if you do not go straight into labour, you will know that this has probably softened and ripened your cervix further.

> Think about the choices that you would like to make about sex at this phase of your pregnancy, considering not only things you *don't* want, but also those you do.
>
> The basis of a mutually satisfying relationship between lovers is good communication. How do you want to indicate your wishes to your partner, in words, gesture and touch? Are there any aspects of each other's sexual feelings and behaviour which it would be helpful to discuss together now – your fears, doubts, hopes and longings?

You can find a good deal more about sex in pregnancy, as well as the sexuality of birth, and sex after the baby comes, in my book *Women's Experience of Sex* (Dorling Kindersley, 1983; Penguin, 1985). The variety of feelings and personal experience in pregnancy is so great that it is impossible to claim that any behaviour is normal or abnormal. You can be sure that, however you feel, there are other women whose experience is very like yours. You are certainly not alone.

For many couples pregnancy is a time of wonder and delight, a vital part of which is the sense of discovery as the woman's body changes, burgeons, ripens. It brings fresh tenderness and passion into their relationship and this excitement and joy prepare them to welcome a new life into the circle of their love.

It is as well that babies do not emerge just a few weeks after they are conceived. A great deal is happening emotionally during pregnancy that needs time to unfold and develop. There are alternatives that need to be explored, about the kind of care that is right for you and your baby and the degree of responsibility you want to take. Sometimes other people assume that you do not *have* any choices, so you have the additional task of making it clear that they do not make decisions *for* you. It is a time when you need to be able to communicate effectively and sometimes stand up to opposition, to learn more about yourself and discover how to work with and express yourself through your body in the most satisfying and harmonious way.

Pregnancy may be uncomfortable – not only physically, but emotionally too. Occasionally you may wish you had never started a baby. Yet this stress can be challenging. It can stimulate fresh thinking and new understanding of yourself and your relationships. It is a period which prepares you to cope with more insight with other stresses and changes which come through the whole of life.

Pregnancy is a learning time. It is a process which, though often stormy – and sometimes tumultuous – encourages an emotional ripening and maturation that give the strength and sensitive awareness to take on responsibility for a new life.

WHAT KIND
OF PRENATAL CARE?

Though it is often taken for granted that seeing a doctor regularly during pregnancy must be a good thing, and that the more medical care a woman has in pregnancy the better, there is very little evidence to support that assumption. It is true that women who have most prenatal visits do not have as many premature babies, but that is because, by definition, premature birth makes pregnancy shorter, so fewer visits are possible.

Seeing a doctor regularly through pregnancy cannot be of any benefit unless the care given is appropriate to a woman's needs. Moreover, in the vast majority of pregnancies the care a woman gives herself, and that which is provided by a partner and other family members, has more significance for her and her baby's well-being than any provided by doctors. It is easy to lose sight of this fact. Basically, prenatal care is not something conferred on a pregnant woman by the medical system. Obstetric services can provide a safety-net, but cannot ensure that a woman has good care throughout her pregnancy.

If you do not want to be merely at the receiving end of medical care, but are keen to look after yourself in the best possible way and get the most effective service from those caring for you, you need to be able to assess what you are offered. In order to do that it is important to think through what you want, if necessary shop around to find it, and also work out how much *personal* responsibility you wish to take for yourself and your baby.

A woman's idea of what she wants from prenatal care may be very different from how an obstetrician sees it. She expects time to talk about worries and fears and wants a good deal of information about the day-to-day experience of pregnancy, how to care for herself, and how to prepare for labour. He – for in most cases it is a 'he' – is usually primarily concerned with screening for a wide range of deviations from the normal, and, according to how she measures up, placing the woman in categories which determine treatment. For many obstetricians, especially those working in large, overcrowded hospitals, it is rather like checking for flaws on a factory production line.

This kind of prenatal care is of relatively recent origin if we see it against the background of history, and how in the past women have had babies in different cultures all over the world. A system of community-based care in which other women are the care-givers has been much more common. Historically, the modern professional organization of care in a medical system staffed by doctors and nurses is an exception rather than the rule. In concentrating exclusively on physical safety, we have lost the emotional support that other women can provide.

The background to care

Midwives have counselled women about nutrition and health, massaged them and given advice on how to prepare for birth from the time of the earliest historical records.[1] There are references to midwives in Genesis. Pregnancy and birth, a female 'mystery' which men knew nothing about, were under the protection of the great mother goddesses, called by many different names – the Earth Mother, the Many Breasted One, the Queen of Light, the Moon Goddess, the Huntress – and later Mary the mother of Jesus.

Women supported each other in birth, shared knowledge which had been handed down from their mothers, and drew on the experience of those who had already borne children. In this way a network of beliefs and practices was created which, in their disintegrated form, we now know only as 'old wives' tales'.[2]

In Third World countries today two systems of prenatal care co-exist. The official one, run by doctors and trained nurses and midwives, is accessible only to a small section of the population. The indigenous system draws on practical skills which women have learned and handed down to each other so as to adjust to that particular environment, and is closely linked with the religion and belief system of the culture. Inevitably, there is conflict between the two. The first employs techniques of measurement and clinical assessment which aim to be objective and identical for every patient. It provides a standard system of care which often treats each woman as if she were merely an ambulant pelvis. On the other hand, there is no doubt that it saves the lives of many babies – and mothers – when pregnancy is abnormal. The second system draws on the power of spiritual forces, and sees the woman in the context of a unique set of social relationships, past and present, with both the living and those who have died, which are thought to affect her and her baby. And it puts special emphasis on psychological conditions which it is important for her and her family to create if she is to have a healthy child and an easy labour.

In Mexico, for instance, it is believed that a pregnant woman must be protected from emotional upset and from people who cause her stress. In the past she used to wear a red cord with which she herself assessed the progress of pregnancy by measuring the growth of the uterus. (In modern clinics much the same procedure is followed, the difference being that professionals do the measuring, not the woman herself.) She took personal responsibility for looking after herself, keeping clean and having daily baths lest the baby get sick, and was familiar with a range of herbal teas to treat minor conditions. Today in Mexico ancient Aztec herbal remedies for urinary infections common in pregnancy are still used – tea brewed with corn tassels or sarsaparilla, for instance.

Throughout the Caribbean the pregnant woman regulates her diet carefully so that her blood is neither too 'hot' nor too 'cold'. She believes that she should have regular exercise in order to be strong for labour and in late pregnancy the local 'nana' (the folk midwife) visits regularly to talk encouragingly to her and to 'shape' the baby by massage and 'make it grow right'.[3]

In South Africa the Zulu woman goes to the door of her hut every morning, where she breathes slowly and deeply for a few minutes as the sun rises, and prays that her baby will grow healthy. Through large parts of Africa it is believed that if labour is to be straightforward a woman must not quarrel with anybody in the weeks preceding and that she and her husband must seek forgiveness for any anger they have for each other. An easy, straightforward labour is seen as dependent upon the right ordering of relationships.

Modern prenatal care

The kind of care we know in the West was started by doctors, not midwives. It was first proposed by Dr Ballantyne of Edinburgh in 1901, though no special clinic was opened until 1915 and a network of clinics was set up later still, at the end of the First World War. The aims of these pioneers were noble: to remove anxiety and discomfort, ensure the early treatment of complications, increase the proportion of normal labours and lower the maternal death and stillbirth rates.

Today the principles of prenatal care have been described by one woman obstetrician,[4] as follows: to identify any abnormality and try to correct or minimize it; attempt to prevent conditions developing which are hazardous for the mother or her baby; if complications occur, select the best time and style of delivery; and help the woman and her partner and family understand and enjoy the birth experience. The objectives have not changed much since the beginning of the last century, but there have been added to them the detection of congenital abnormalities, and preparation for childbirth and parenthood. Most recently, concern has developed over what happens even before conception and with the effects of social deprivation and poverty: birth is much more dangerous for the babies of poor mothers than for those of the comfortably off.

Doctors are learning that social factors have greater influence on pregnancy and its outcome than anything they can do.[5] In Britain, for example, 16 babies in every 1,000 whose fathers are in semi-skilled or unskilled occupations die at or around the time of birth compared with 11 of those whose fathers are in the professional classes.[6]

In all Western countries the highest rates of death and sickness occur in the babies of working-class mothers and of recent immigrants from Third World countries. And a woman born in Pakistan but having a baby in the West is more than twice as likely as a British-born woman to lose her baby at or around birth.[7]

Such factors as lack of education, poor housing, inadequate nutrition, unemployment and working in a toxic environment can all adversely affect the well-being of the mother and her baby. The kind of care provided today does little or nothing to reduce the impact of social pressures like these which put many women under physical and emotional stress during pregnancy, and are a threat to them and their unborn babies. Poverty is the major cause of baby deaths – and no amount of micro-chip technology can make up for that.

But it is not just a question of babies dying – perinatal mortality. Many babies are born prematurely, of low birth-weight, sick, or in some other way handicapped – perinatal morbidity. In the words of a sociologist, Ann Oakley: 'Reducing social disadvantage – whether in the form of poor housing, inadequate disposable income, deficient diet, or whatever – is not a different issue from the issue of improving the perinatal mortality and morbidity, but the same issue.'[8]

Problems in high-tech care

Right at the beginning of this chapter I pointed out that everyone more or less assumes that there ought to be more prenatal care. It is put forward as an example of the best kind of preventive medicine.

Yet when we get down to measuring its success and cost-effectiveness, little data is available. In fact, prenatal care has grown piecemeal from the last century, bits being added to it over the years without proper assessment, and without anybody finding out at what phase of pregnancy specific kinds of care are appropriate or to which women different elements of care should be offered.[9] It is taken for granted that it must be a good thing, however complicated it becomes, whatever the cost, and whatever the effects on the pregnant woman and her family. Care-givers, often with the best will in the world, use their authority to indoctrinate the pregnant woman with the idea that she should passively undergo any and every investigation – however stressful to her – for the sake of her baby. She is, after all, the container for the fetus, and society demands of her that she submit to whatever screening procedures can enable obstetricians to know more about exactly what is happening inside the uterus – that tantalizingly locked cupboard which, by a seemingly inexorable process of advancement in science, is becoming more and more like those plastic see-through snap-shut cases in the models of the female body used to demonstrate our reproductive anatomy.

Technology has enabled doctors to introduce a whole range of new screening tests into prenatal care. But these have produced new problems. One is that of the *false positive* diagnosis, and the unnecessary intervention that often takes place because of it. A false positive occurs when, as a result of a test which gives incorrect information or is misinterpreted, a diagnosis is made which attaches to a woman a disease or 'high risk' label. That label sticks even if other tests show later that nothing is wrong after all. The anxiety it produces often remains with the woman and those caring for her, and this may affect their actions later and lead to unnecessary intervention when she goes into labour, too.

One common false positive is the diagnosis, following a sonar scan at 16 weeks, of a low-lying placenta, which may mean a Caesarean section. But a low-lying placenta is very common in the first half of pregnancy, and as the uterus enlarges later in pregnancy the placenta is often found to be in a good position. Or, again following a scan, a woman may be warned that the baby is not growing in the uterus, but in spite of this later gives birth to an eight-pounder. One study revealed that 2.5 false positive diagnoses of intra-uterine growth retardation (IGR) were made for every one correctly diagnosed.[10]

Doctors, on the whole, do not worry so much about false positives as about false negatives. They prefer to err on the side of over-diagnosis of problems than to miss signs of malfunction or disease, and the thought of failing to note evidence that a physiological process is going wrong triggers a great deal of anxiety and, especially in North America, worry about possible litigation. Yet the consequence of false positive diagnosis can be catastrophic for the woman – unnecessary hospitalization, induction of labour and Caesarean section, for instance – and a baby born before it is ready is exposed to the danger of prematurity.

False negatives are obviously dangerous, since they suggest that everything is all right when, in fact, something is wrong. They have the effect of switching off the warning light which clinical judgement and human experience turned on. Although assessment of fetal growth results in more false positives than false negatives, a good many instances of intra-uterine growth retardation are not revealed by standard prenatal care. In one study doctors suspected it in only 44 per cent of women who later had low-birth-weight babies.[11] Obviously diagnoses of intra-uterine growth retardation are very much a hit-and-miss affair!

When tests are performed the woman is rarely asked what she knows, and what she says is usually ignored. Another kind of false negative can result when the baby's heart-beat is recorded in pregnancy and no abnormality is indicated, though the woman herself realizes that she is no longer noticing any movements, and after some days the baby dies. It is a rare occurrence, but one which shatters confidence in high-technology care. The mother felt that something was wrong – but nobody asked her what *she* knew about her baby and doctors relied on technology instead.

Prenatal care, even when given conscientiously – and it isn't always – and even when professionals are up to date with knowledge – and they aren't always – can be ineffective, and sometimes dangerous.

Some people think the lesson to be learned from this is to have still more routine investigations and more sophisticated technology. Others believe there is a great deal to be learned from women themselves, and that what a woman knows about her body and the way in which she can be in touch with her baby inside should form a major theme of care through pregnancy.

Yet medical care usually makes a woman distrust her own first-hand experience and her awareness of her baby. Her medical records present the sole validated reality.

The only things we are supposed to 'know' about our health and the progress of pregnancy are those which can be recorded and measured by observers and entered in charts and case-notes. Everything else is considered irrelevant. An elaborate system of procedures has been developed, one effect of which is to deny women knowledge they can have about themselves.

Many of these routines have become heavily ritualized – part of a symbolic process by which a woman is turned into a patient. One example of a ceremony of this kind is the regular weighing at each visit – as if she were not capable of keeping track of her weight at home. These rituals are employed routinely on all women, though they can be shown to be useful only in certain specific 'high-risk' cases. Ultrasound is also used in a ritual manner, though the benefits of routine ultrasound investigations have never been scientifically demonstrated. It has become an 'insurance' against disaster.

You do not *have* to agree to any interventions. If your doctor cannot provide you with evidence that a screening procedure or a treatment is going to do you any good, you are not only free to refuse it, but may be wise to do so.

The authors of a midwifery textbook suggest that the label of 'high-risk' ought to be replaced by a different concept – that of 'levels of care'.[12] Some women need more concentrated care than others or care of a different kind. As we shall see later, risk-oriented prenatal screening often leads to care inappropriate to a woman's needs and harmful intervention such as unnecessary induction of labour.

Though doctors treat pregnancy as a medical condition, it really is not. Eighty per cent of women have completely normal pregnancies and labours. Twenty per cent are at some special risk. But only half of these are discovered to be at risk during pregnancy. The others' problems are only recognized during labour. So at present the whole system of prenatal care works efficiently for only 10 per cent of women.

Even when prenatal care is accurate, the way a woman *feels* about the care she gets and how she is treated by doctors is of paramount importance. For pregnancy and birth are bio-social processes. They do not simply operate like a process in mechanical engineering, though obstetric textbooks often give this impression. A frequent effect of prenatal care is to drain away a woman's self-confidence and, through medicalization of the whole experience of pregnancy and birth, to deprive her of autonomy and make her feel inadequate, helpless – and often guilty – because she feels that if she really cares for her baby she should not mind being treated like this.

When a woman becomes a patient she also tends to be isolated from the help and emotional support of other women. In the past the announcement of a pregnancy was an occasion for reinforcing solidarity among women in the family and neighbourhood. In medieval times a woman starting labour called together her 'God sibs' (a word which later became corrupted to 'gossips') to care for and comfort her during child-birth, bring food and strong drink, and have what amounted to a cele-bratory birth feast. The men might grumble about it, but they were expected to leave the house and fend for themselves. Birth was women's business! Similarly, in colonial America pregnancy and birth were pri-marily social processes based on reciprocity, women caring for each other and giving practical help and emotional support.

In contrast, today a woman is taught to put her faith in medical advisers and distrust all that other women can teach her, which is dis-missed, in one obstetrician's words, as a 'cartload of rubbish'.[13] He warns expectant mothers not to listen to 'wicked women with their malicious, lying tongues'. The ideal pregnancy patient should, according to this view, be the doctor's obedient pupil, with ears only for his instructions and a willingness to follow them unquestioningly.

Prenatal clinics are so poorly organized in many countries of the West that some probably do more harm than good. Those women who do not have a private obstetrician or an individual midwife who cares for them throughout, and who attend large hospital clinics, are exposed to the risks which come from lack of continuity in care and the muddle and confusion which results from that. They say things like: 'There was a conveyor belt feeling. I saw a different doctor each time.' 'Treatment was impersonal. Confusion over dates was never resolved. Twice they told me I ought to be induced.' (The baby would have arrived five weeks early!) 'The clinic was extremely bureaucratic. We were constantly being herded from one line to another. I came away from each visit in tears, feeling that motherhood was being degraded.'

In a hospital clinic a woman is the passive object of management. Fed into the system, her progress through it from point to point is controlled as if she had no wishes of her own. Large hospitals are often a long way from where those they are intended to serve live or work, so that women have an arduous journey to attend. Then they have to wait, for an hour, two hours, three – sometimes even more – in surroundings which are often extremely uncomfortable and depressing. In almost any large clinic a visitor can see rows of women sitting waiting for the doctor. The assumption is that though the obstetrician should never have to wait for a woman, it is acceptable for a woman to wait to see an obstetrician. The doctor's time is always more valuable than the patient's.

Few hospitals provide anything for women to do *except* wait. Facilities for childcare are usually absent and toddlers become fractious and weary. The clinics are also often overcrowded and the atmosphere is that of a badly managed cattle market. Women tend to get conflicting information and advice.

Any discussion with the obstetrician is restricted to a couple of minutes. Many women see this as the whole point of the visit and their planning and waiting are directed towards this moment. They are desperately disappointed when they are in and out of the examination room in a matter of minutes and have no opportunity for asking questions or voicing their anxieties. Instead they find themselves lying flat on their backs, pants off and exposed from the waist down, being prodded and poked while all they can see is the hair in the doctor's nostrils. This done, the doctor often disappears to see the next patient and the woman is told that she can get up and dress now.

When that kind of thing happens to you, and you get emotional, it is easy to feel that there must be something wrong with *you*, *other* women do not seem near to tears. You blame yourself for being over-sensitive or expecting special treatment. When talking with pregnant women I am often struck by the way in which they feel trapped in a situation they are powerless to influence and in which they are completely isolated. Yet this experience is so general that you are not really alone with it. It is worth talking with other women about how you feel and seeing if there is anything you can do to change the situation.

Many care-givers are concerned about what is happening, too. Women sociologists have stressed the negative experience that women have of prenatal care and have shown how anxious it makes them, and some doctors and midwives are well aware that things need changing and may welcome any help you can give them in order to effect change.[14]

In clinics like these, doctors, nurses and midwives are also under stress. When a great many women converge on an overcrowded clinic within a short period of time there is bound to be anxiety for staff as well as mothers, since they are under pressure to keep the flow through and often feel frustrated and guilty because it is impossible to give adequate care. Their work is fragmented and task-oriented rather than person-oriented, with the result that they, as well as the women, feel as if they are on an assembly line.

Yet private obstetrics, though it offers more continuity of care and more comfortable – sometimes even luxurious – conditions, still does not ensure that you get the kind of care you want. All too often a woman is coaxed along by an obstetrician who is trying to reassure her, but who does not really intend to allow her choice, except in trivial matters. Women wanting natural childbirth often encounter filibustering and insincerity, and sometimes outright deceit, from obstetricians who want 'the little woman' to take them on trust. 'You can have your baby hanging from the chandelier as far as I'm concerned,' (another version is 'standing on your head') 'but if you are in too much pain I'll have to intervene.' 'Of *course* you can have a natural birth. *All* birth is natural . . .' The same authoritarianism, the same paternalism that controls women in a large hospital clinic is hidden behind the face of the salesmanship inherent in private obstetrics.

Midwives and obstetricians

You do not have to have an obstetrician. In many areas you can choose to have some, most or all of your care from a midwife. She may work independently, as in the Netherlands, as one of a team of midwives, or with a family practitioner who does obstetrics, as community midwives do in Britain. Trained midwives are able to take full responsibility for care in pregnancy, at the birth and afterwards. They can call in other help when they think it is needed. In practice, though, in many European countries this professional responsibility is being removed from midwives, so that increasingly they work as members of hospital-based teams headed by obstetricians. This means that more and more they take their instructions from obstetricians and in some countries – Italy and Germany, for example – midwives are becoming like North American obstetric nurses, assistants to obstetricians. In Britain, too, more than 75 per cent of those midwives who work in teaching hospitals are supposed to refer to doctors about the conduct of normal deliveries – though in practice this often does not happen. Over 90 per cent of midwives who work in hospital clinics are not required to use their skills and judgement to the extent to which they are qualified.[15] They are used as receptionists and chaperones, or to test urine and weigh patients. It is not surprising that in Britain only one of every five midwives who qualifies actually practises, and of these most leave midwifery within five years. Even so, around 80 per cent of babies are delivered by midwives, and within the National Health Service doctors usually do only the complicated deliveries.

Because things have become so bad, midwives are now organizing themselves to redefine the role of the midwife and make a clear distinction between midwifery and obstetrics. There is a strong and growing movement of 'radical' midwifery – a term which means literally 'going back to the roots'.

In North America, where the medical profession forced it into virtual extinction in the early years of the century, there is now a rebirth of midwifery. Many women prefer to be cared for by a midwife. Yet in the USA many states, and in Canada provinces, refuse to recognize midwifery or to register women as midwives. As a result 'lay' midwives are practising, mostly illegally, though there are some places where they can be registered. Sometimes they are called 'empirical' or 'practical' midwives. In those areas where midwifery is illegal, both lay midwives and nurse-midwives (who go through training as a nurse before they start their midwife training) live continually under the threat of possible prosecution and imprisonment for 'practising medicine without a licence'. Some lay midwives are excellent. Others have suffered because there is no systematic training. Similarly, some nurse-midwives who are working closely with obstetricians are more like doctors than other midwives. Others are skilled in supporting the natural process of labour. In North America midwifery is almost synonymous with home birth, since in most states midwives are not allowed to deliver babies in hospital. If they do catch babies it is because the obstetrician did not arrive on time, or occasionally because they have been given another name, such as 'extended role nurses', as part of a research programme to compare the safety of midwife-attended birth with doctor-attended birth. Many midwives also work in out-of-hospital birth centres where birth is treated as a normal life process and there is little or no intervention.

It may not be easy for you to get one-to-one care from a midwife. And if you want care that is different from that on standard offer you may have to seek far and be extraordinarily persistent.

In considering the type of care you want during pregnancy you will obviously have to think ahead to the birth, too, because this may involve the same people and your choice of care-givers for the birth will almost certainly limit those available to look after you during pregnancy. You need to bear both in mind at the same time.

Though there are vast differences between practices in different countries, and in the United States, for example, between the West Coast and the Mid-West, and rural and urban areas, in general the following differences exist between midwives and obstetricians:

A midwife	*An obstetrician*
Is almost invariably a woman. (Midwifery is open to men, but very few choose it as a career.)	Is usually a man (though more women are going into obstetrics now).
May be a specialist in natural birth.	Is a specialist in dealing with things that go wrong.
May work independently or as part of a small non-specialized group.	Heads a team in which there are other specialists – e.g., a neonatologist, anaesthetist, radiologist, physiotherapist.
May not have easy access to specialized equipment if she does not work in a fully equipped hospital.	Has access to specialized equipment – e.g., electronic fetal monitoring, ultrasound, X-ray, certain lab tests.

That list is obviously over-simplified and it is important for you to find out the situation in your own area if you want to make choices between alternative kinds of care.

Look at the list again and when you have found out about conditions in your own area alter it as necessary to apply more accurately to the situation there. If you can make personal contact, add information about particular midwives and doctors whom you are considering. Allow a column for each midwife and doctor about whom you have information.

If you can discover rates of intervention – for instance, what percentage of women have a perineal shave, suppositories or an enema, an intravenous drip set up, labour augmented with oxytocin, artificial rupture of membranes, episiotomy, or an operative delivery, include these facts in your list, too. (These subjects are discussed in Chapter 11.) You will then be in a better position to decide on an appropriate care-giver or, if you have one already, to consider the advantages and disadvantages of this person compared with others and decide whether you want to change.

The preliminary visit

Your first visit to a doctor or midwife may be a preliminary one to see if you can get on together and if you share the same view of childbirth. You may not want to make a firm decision before you have had such a meeting. In some care systems it is difficult to arrange any personal contact like this and you are expected to go on trust and simply hand yourself over to professionals, relying on them to do what is best for you. If this is how you are expected to act, be especially careful to shop around first, talking to other women who have had babies recently. Ask local childbirth organizations and teachers for their advice. You may need to do some quite complicated detective work. This is an important decision. You would make careful enquiries about a hairdresser before letting him give you a new hair-style, or an architect before asking her to design you a house. You have the right to be at least as careful about whoever you choose to look after you in pregnancy and birth.

Though you will obviously want to assess whether your care-giver understands your approach to childbirth and is sympathetic towards it, avoid going with a list of demands. Statements put in terms of 'do's and don'ts' are invariably over-simplified and do not take account of what may happen to make you want to modify your views. The important thing is whether you can communicate and work together well. On the other hand, you need to explain exactly where your priorities lie. Otherwise there may be serious misunderstandings. Do not be fobbed off by soothing noises and reassurance. Get it right out in the open.

It is useful to have some written notes you can refer to so that you remember to discuss the aspects of care which are most important to you. Chapter 10 may help you say what you want and negotiate effectively, and the last two sections of the book can give you some idea of the different styles of birth to consider.

So far as the place of birth is concerned, bear in mind that a doctor may not always be the best person to advise you about where to have the baby – and certainly is not the only one. You need to talk with other women about this and find out what they liked or disliked about the places where they gave birth. Childbirth education organizations and women's health centres can help you too.

The first consultation

Once you have decided on your care-giver, the first consultation, or in Britain, the booking clinic, is important because you are likely to have more opportunity to talk than at subsequent visits. A doctor or midwife takes your 'history' on this occasion. This includes details about your own health – and any previous pregnancies and births – and, if the information is available, that of the baby's father and both your families. You are given a complete physical examination. Your height is measured and you are weighed. A sample of blood is taken to measure the level of haemoglobin (the oxygen-carrying part of the red blood cell), find out whether you are Rhesus positive or negative and test for syphilis. If you are in a vulnerable group you may also be tested to see if you are a carrier of sickle cell anaemia or Tay-Sachs syndrome. You are asked to give a midstream specimen of urine, too, so that it can be checked for bacteria and for sugar, which might indicate diabetes.

A vaginal examination is usually done to assess the size of your uterus and check it against the date of your last menstrual period. A cervical smear may also be taken to test for pre-cancerous cells in the cervix. If you have any vaginal discharge the doctor can take a swab and test it for thrush (candida) and sexually transmitted disease. You should be offered a chest X-ray if you come from an area where TB is common.

Another test that is often performed at this or the next visit involves measuring the level of alpha fetoprotein (AFP) in your blood. If it is high there is an increased risk of the baby having a neural tube defect (a central nervous system handicap such as spina bifida, in which a part of the spinal cord protrudes from the back). This test cannot be done before 16 weeks (from the first day of your last period). Women over 35 are usually also offered amniocentesis, which tests the water in which the baby floats to discover whether or not it suffers from a range of conditions, including chromosomal disorders such as Down's syndrome, and neural tube defects. Again, this test cannot be done until 16 to 18 weeks. There is no cure for these conditions but you can choose to have the pregnancy terminated. Although it may be too early to have these tests done at your first prenatal visit, it is a good idea to discuss them then and to let your doctor know how you feel about them.

Many obstetricians perform routine ultrasound examinations at 16 weeks – some earlier than this – in order to check your dates. Some make regular ultrasound checks to record the baby's growth right through pregnancy. Since there is no evidence that routine use of ultrasound is of any benefit, you may have your own ideas about this, too, and if so, you should discuss them with the doctor.

Tests Done at the First Visit

TEST	WHY IT IS DONE
Weight	Have base from which to assess weight gain during pregnancy.
Blood	Ascertain blood group. Reveal possible Rhesus incompatibility. Measure haemoglobin. Check for sexually transmitted disease so that it can be treated.
Urine	Check for presence of bacteria, so bladder infection can be treated. Check for sugar, possible symptom of gestational diabetes.
If it is your first baby, nipple examination	See if there are likely to be breastfeeding difficulties because of inverted nipples. (This is unnecessary, because once you can get a baby well fixed, the baby shapes the nipples beautifully.)
Palpation of abdomen	Feel size of uterus and level of top of uterus.
Possible vaginal examination	Confirm pregnancy. Take swab in case of discharge so that infection can be treated. Do cervical smear to check for pre-cancerous condition of cervix.
Blood pressure	Find base level against which any later rise can be measured.

At this first visit you should also discuss where you are going to have your baby – home or hospital or in some kind of alternative birth centre. If you decide on hospital you may want to consider a birthing room in the hospital if it is available. The range of options varies in different countries. But if you are to choose between alternatives you want to know exactly what is available and the pros and cons of each. If you find you cannot come to an agreement about this it is not too late to change your care-giver.

Visits usually take place every four weeks until 28 weeks, then every two weeks till 36 weeks and each week from then on. For most women –

those who start pregnancy in good health and continue to feel well – this number of visits to an obstetrician before 36 weeks is pointless.

A pregnant woman is perfectly capable of charting her own weight gain and, using a clinical dipstick, of checking her urine for the presence of protein (which is one symptom of developing pre-eclamptic toxaemia, a metabolic disorder of pregnancy) and for sugar. What many women feel they need most, but cannot find, is the chance to talk to knowledgeable and understanding women who have first-hand experience of pregnancy and birth.

Raised blood pressure and pre-eclamptic toxaemia (PET)

You will see that many routine pregnancy tests are concerned with the detection of pre-eclampsia. This is important because you may feel perfectly well and not realize that anything is wrong. Pre-eclampsia leads to reduction in blood supply to the placenta, the baby's life-support system. The symptoms are raised blood pressure, albumen in the urine, marked oedema (retention of fluids under the skin) and sudden weight gain. Raised blood pressure (hypertension) can exist by itself or as one element in PET. Mild pre-eclampsia in the last few weeks occurs in approximately 25 per cent of all pregnancies.[16] It is so frequent as to be normal. But pre-eclampsia which starts earlier in pregnancy (before 36 weeks), or which is severe – when blood pressure is higher than 160/100 – even with late onset, is serious. This severe kind occurs in only one fifth of all cases of pre-eclampsia. If the diastolic pressure – the lowest level to which blood pressure falls between heartbeats – goes up to 110 or more, or there is albumen in the urine *and* the diastolic pressure is 90 or more, or if the woman actually develops eclampsia and has fits, there is a risk that the baby may die.[17]

Blood pressure readings are recorded with the systolic pressure – the highest pressure reached during a heartbeat – as an upper figure and the diastolic pressure underneath it. The upper figure changes at different times of the day and when you are feeling angry or anxious. If you have to rush to get to your appointment or drive through heavy traffic, it will probably go up. The lower figure is the important one.

For a blood pressure reading to be accurate you should be relaxed. It is often difficult to feel at ease when you visit your doctor, especially if you are worried that your blood pressure may be up. The expression 'white-

Tests Done Every Two Weeks

TEST	WHY IT IS DONE	HOW TO DO IT YOURSELF
Weight	Assess growth of baby and reveal any sudden weight gain, a possible symptom of pre-eclampsia.	Weigh yourself at about the same time of day, wearing similar clothing. After the first 3 months some women put on weight in swoops and starts. Most weeks there is a steady rise of 200–400 g, with a total weight gain of up to 12 kg. The baby can still be a good weight if you gain less or more than this.
Urine	Check for presence of bacteria, so bladder infection can be treated.	Cannot be done yourself. Specimen must be sent to a lab.
	Check for sugar, possible symptom of gestational diabetes.	Use dip-sticks, which change colour to indicate presence of albumen or sugar. You can buy them from a women's health centre or chemist.
	Check for presence of albumen (protein) one symptom of pre-eclampsia.	
Blood pressure	Check whether there is any rise – sharp rise is one symptom of pre-eclampsia	Get a friend to help you, using a sphygmomanometer (blood pressure gauge).
Palpation of abdomen	Feel size of uterus and level of top of uterus. Feel position and size of baby	See pp. 184–7. If you would like to learn how to do it yourself, ask your midwife to show you.
Fetal heart monitoring	Check baby's heart rate – normally 120–160 beats per minute.	Use a long stethoscope or get a friend to listen using the cardboard cylinder from a lavatory paper roll. Listen for 15 seconds and then multiply by four.
In late pregnancy also: Possible vaginal examination	Reveal position of baby's head and whether cervix is ripe for labour.	Best done by a doctor or midwife.

coat hypertension' has been coined to describe what happens when blood pressure shoots up in the presence of a doctor.[18] Your blood pressure is likely to be lower at home than in hospital.[19] It will vary at different times of the day and is usually lowest first thing in the morning. Single blood pressure readings are unreliable.[20] Some heart specialists suggest that the most accurate records come when patients take their own serial blood pressure measurements at home, or when a friend or someone in the family helps them do so. In some areas where community midwives still come to the home for prenatal visits, pregnant women often notice that their blood pressure is higher when taken by the general practitioner, higher still when done in the hospital and lowest when measured by the community midwife at home. So if your blood pressure is slightly up at the end of pregnancy, as it is for many women, and there is concern that it may be rising, you may want to borrow or buy a sphygmomanometer (blood-pressure gauge) and learn how to measure it yourself at home.

Women nearing the end of pregnancy who have pre-eclampsia are usually advised to have labour induced. Those with marginally raised blood pressure are often told that they are developing pre-eclampsia and thus ought to have labour induced. It is best not to agree to induction of labour unless your blood pressure is dangerously high.

There are all sorts of ideas about what causes pre-eclampsia: not only poor nutrition, as we have seen in Chapter 4, but also being tense and under pressure, poverty – and our whole Western way of living. It certainly seems to be a physiological stress disease. A woman is more likely to develop it if her body has to adapt to cope with a twin pregnancy, for example, or if she is especially young or old. First-time mothers (primigravidae) are also more likely to get it than those having subsequent babies (multigravidae).

If symptoms of pre-eclampsia are diagnosed a doctor will want to admit you to hospital for bed-rest and may advise drug treatment. Diuretics, drugs which promote the flow of urine, are often used since they lower blood pressure. There have been 11 randomized trials of diuretics in pregnancy which show that there is no reliable evidence of the value of this treatment.[21]

The other drugs used are beta blockers, which block the action of adrenalin on the heart. There have been few controlled trials of these, though one systematic study with follow-up when the babies were a year old revealed no major disadvantages.[22] But it has to be remembered that there is rapid development of a child's central nervous system throughout the first three years of life and some problems may not crop up till much later. In view of this, some researchers believe that 'follow-up until the age of 7 years is mandatory before a drug given to the mother during pregnancy can be considered even relatively safe'.[23] Doctors are under great pressure from drug companies to employ these drugs, but their use at present is, on the whole, more or less unevaluated and uncontrolled.[24]

If pre-eclampsia becomes severe and rest in bed does nothing to reduce it, there may be no effective treatment other than induction of labour. There comes a point when the baby is better out than in.

Since one in four of all pregnant women are classified by doctors as having some form of pre-eclampsia, even though mild, it is sensible to think ahead about what you would want if you developed any symptoms. Talk about this with your partner or with someone else who could take over your responsibilities and make a plan of action together. Jot down the rough outline of this in your notebook. It will help to look at your life-style and see how you can simplify it and cut out stress. If you are planning to have a break from work outside the home, for example, the time to do so is when you get the earliest symptoms of pre-eclampsia, rather than waiting till it is severe and then having to go into hospital. Your partner, or someone else, will need to take over household chores so that you can rest as much as you can. The relaxation you learn in childbirth classes, breathing slowly and fully and relaxing a little more with each breath *out*, helps bring down blood pressure. Since raised blood pressure tends to occur at a stage of pregnancy when sleep is most likely to be disturbed, you may want to try a natural sleep-inducer consisting of amino acids – tryptophan. This is available from health-food stores. If you do not have to wake several times in the night to empty your bladder, a milk drink before you sleep can help. At the end of pregnancy you may sleep better on your own.

Outline a plan of action in case your blood pressure should go up after 36 weeks or there are other symptoms of possible pre-eclampsia. To be forewarned is to be forearmed.

Note any questions you might want to ask.

Make a list of people you could call on for help and the arrangements you would need to make.

You may be told that you will be booked for an epidural when labour starts in order to lower your blood pressure. If you are coping with contractions do not be persuaded by this, as an epidural has no effect on maximum levels of blood pressure – the ones that matter. Whether or not to have an epidural should be your own decision.

The anxiety many women feel in pregnancy cannot be explained away by saying that they are in an emotionally vulnerable state and that it is all a matter of hormones. When a baby is coming, social and economic problems that did not seem daunting before can become overwhelming because you are taking on responsibility for a new life. It may be important to discuss stresses in relationships, worries about financial matters or living conditions, or fears about the birth or how you are going to manage afterwards, with someone who understands and can help you reduce these stresses. If they cannot be removed, you have the opportunity of working out ways of coping with them better.

DECIDING ABOUT SPECIAL TESTS

The border-line between routine tests in pregnancy and special screening done if there is reason to suspect abnormality is a fuzzy one. In many countries an increasing number of tests designed to detect slight and unimportant deviations from the normal, on the one hand, and rare conditions which can have serious consequences, on the other, are being introduced into routine care. Knowing about them, what they are and why they are done, can help you decide whether or not you want to have them. The choice is yours. Even if it has been proved conclusively that a test is valuable, you still have a right to refuse it. No one can compel you to agree to any medical intervention whatsoever.

Some of these screening procedures entail further analyses of the blood which is taken as a matter of course at the first visit or soon after that. Others involve an extra blood test or other kind of investigation.

Blood glucose monitoring

It is very important that a woman with diabetes has regular monitoring of blood glucose concentrations during pregnancy. Previous obstetric practice has often been to deliver the baby early by inducing labour at about 37 weeks, but it is now being shown that with careful control of blood sugar it can be safe for women to wait to go into spontaneous labour. Women can monitor their own blood glucose concentrations effectively at home. When they do there are fewer hospital admissions and a reduced Caesarean section rate, and the babies are in better condition.[1] This is one situation where scrupulous monitoring through pregnancy is extremely important and where women themselves, instead of being merely at the receiving end of prenatal care, can take personal responsibility and an active role in looking after themselves.

AFP blood test

The level of alpha fetoprotein – a substance produced by the baby's liver and gastrointestinal tract – in the mother's blood can be measured to find out if the baby is likely to have a neural tube defect – a handicap resulting from failure of the spinal cord to form correctly or to close.

Screening is done between 16 and 18 weeks. A higher than usual level of AFP suggests that the baby may have a congenital handicap involving the spinal cord. In some places this screening procedure is done routinely on all mothers.

In others it is done only if, because of family history or because a woman has already had a baby with a congenital handicap, there is cause for concern. There are many arguments for and against routine screening. Some people say that if a woman is not told that her blood is to be used for this purpose it should not be done. Others say that to introduce the possibility of congenital handicap, with no evidence that it exists, is to sow seeds of anxiety in the pregnant woman's mind. In some areas doctors point to a low incidence of abnormality which can be revealed by AFP testing and therefore consider it an unnecessary and costly procedure. Only 10 per cent of women who have a raised AFP level in their blood and go on to have amniocentesis actually have babies suffering from central nervous system abnormalities, so there is a very wide margin of error.

One reason for this is that AFP levels are raised if a woman has her dates wrong. They roughly double every five weeks in the second three months of pregnancy, and the gap between normal and very high levels is greatest between the sixteenth and eighteenth weeks. If you are further on in pregnancy than you think, the AFP level will be higher than expected. A twin pregnancy will also push up the AFP level. If you have viral hepatitis it will be raised too.

In North America the rate of neural tube defects is one in 1,000 pregnancies, whereas in Britain it is a good deal higher – 4.5 for every 1,000 pregnancies. This is one reason why AFP screening is more usual in Britain than in the USA. However, testing cannot completely rule out the possibility that a baby may have a neural tube defect.[2]

If you ask for a blood AFP test, or if your obstetrician advises it, bear in mind that if the level is up this will cause a lot of anxiety until you have amniocentesis, and then for another four weeks or more until the results come. Think ahead to how you would want to cope and the support you might need. Many women find that an understanding woman friend who has been through it all herself is a great help. Many talk it through with their partners and face it together. Whatever happens, do not try to push it to the back of your mind and pretend that it has not happened. It is better to bring the anxiety out into the open and acknowledge it, while at the same time keeping busy with other things and living life as fully as possible.

Amniocentesis

Amniocentesis is a test of the amniotic fluid in which the baby floats. It cannot be done until 16 to 18 weeks because until then there is insufficient fluid. A needle is introduced through the mother's abdominal wall into the uterus to draw off a sample of fluid so that it can be examined to show the level of alpha fetoprotein (AFP) and fetal cells in it can be grown in a culture to reveal a range of chromosomal abnormalities, including Down's syndrome, and spina bifida and anencephaly.

If amniocentesis reveals that the baby suffers from a congenital handicap the mother decides whether or not to have an abortion, something which most women have thought about in advance of having the test – and, indeed, some say there is no point in having it because they would not agree to abortion.

To be able to predict which babies will be handicapped or may die from a congenital abnormality is a major scientific advance. For women at special risk of bearing handicapped babies because certain kinds of abnormality run in their or their partner's families, or because they are in an 'at risk' age-group, it may be an enormous relief to know that they can abort an affected fetus. The equation is different for every woman, and her personal feelings, which are often very mixed, must be an important part of any decision she makes. It is not something that can be worked out with a slide-rule.

The US National Genetic Foundation advises that the following women should have amniocentesis:

- All women over 35.
- Any woman who knows, as the result of a genetic test, that she and the father of her baby carry the same gene for congenital disease.
- Those who have already borne a child with a biochemical or developmental disorder which can be diagnosed prenatally.
- Women from ethnic groups at special risk of a genetic disorder. Black women should be tested for sickle cell anaemia; those of

Mediterranean ancestry for thalassaemia, a haemoglobin abnormality; and descendants of Central and Eastern European Jews for Tay-Sachs disease, an enzyme deficiency disease which leads to brain damage.

● Women with diabetes or PET who have been advised to have an induced labour or an elective (planned) Caesarean section if the baby will be premature should have third-trimester amniocentesis.

Amniocentesis also reveals the sex of the baby – relevant if there are sex-linked diseases, such as haemophilia or Duchenne muscular dystrophy, where girls carry the disorder but do not suffer from it. In societies where girls have little value and where the birth of sons is of paramount importance female babies may be aborted following amniocentesis. Sometimes a father insists on abortion though the woman wants to bear the child. The new power to discover what is going on inside the uterus raises ethical dilemmas and must bring with it new responsibility to wield that power wisely.

If you have amniocentesis you may want to know the sex of your baby, but not all doctors will give that information. This is partly because they believe that women may seek abortion of babies of the unwanted sex. Women themselves often do not want to know the sex because they feel it is more natural not to know and prefer a baby to be a surprise. Others want to have all the information they can. But, either way, women should have the *right* to know. Whatever can be learnt from amniocentesis should not be in a medically restricted category of knowledge.

In 1985 it first became possible to identify with 99-per-cent reliability fetuses which would develop cystic fibrosis, a disease which leads to severe digestive disturbances and damages the lungs. A child suffering from it has a life expectancy of only 20 years. But at this stage it is still not possible to predict which parents carry the defective gene, so the test can help only those women who have already had a child with cystic fibrosis.

Later on in pregnancy an analysis of amniotic fluid can also reveal whether the fetal lungs are mature and whether, if born at that stage, the newborn baby is likely to develop respiratory distress syndrome (RDS). This is important information if a baby is very premature. But even then results are not 100-per-cent accurate and many babies diagnosed as not ready for independent life breathe well after delivery.[3]

Amniocentesis cannot guarantee that any baby will be perfect, since it only screens for a range of specific handicaps. Research by the Royal College of Obstetricians and Gynaecologists on late abortions showed that

Rates of Down's syndrome in live births by maternal age from 35 years

WOMAN'S AGE	INCIDENCE	WOMAN'S AGE	INCIDENCE
35	1 in 365	43	1 in 50
36	,, 290	44	,, 40
37	,, 225	45	,, 32
38	,, 180	46	,, 25
39	,, 140	47	,, 20
40	,, 109	48	,, 15
41	,, 85	49	,, 12
42	,, 70		

From J. Simpson, 'Antenatal diagnosis of cytogenetic abnormalities', *Seminars in Perinatology*, 4: 3 (1980), 168

when they were done because amniocentesis revealed a raised AFP level, 6.5 per cent of fetuses were not handicapped in any way and of the rest 15 per cent did not have open neural tube defects. (This means they had very mild spina bifida which would not have caused any problem.)[4] So there is the possibility that a normal baby could be aborted on the off-chance that it was abnormal. This is another of the ethical dilemmas associated with amniocentesis.

Rates of chromosome abnormalities at amniocentesis in 5-year stages

WOMAN'S AGE	INCIDENCE	WOMAN'S AGE	INCIDENCE
25	1 in 527	40	1 in 73
30	,, 476	45	,, 23
35	,, 204		

From E. B. Hook and D. K. Cross, 'Estimated rates of clinically significant cytogenetic abnormality (other than Down's syndrome)', *American Journal of Human Genetics*, 31, (1979) 136a

Note: A number of babies with chromosome abnormalities are miscarried. So the rate discovered at amniocentesis is higher than that of babies actually born with these handicaps. At 35, for example, there is a 1 in 222 chance of a baby being born with such an abnormality, compared with a 1 in 204 chance at the time of amniocentesis; at 40 a 1 in 83 chance compared with 1 in 73 at amniocentesis; and at 45 1 in 30 compared with 1 in 23 at amniocentesis.

How amniocentesis is done

Amniocentesis takes place in a small room which looks rather like an operating theatre, with a trolley packed with phials, bottles and packets of swabs and with an ultrasound screen which looks like a TV. The test must be done under sterile conditions, or infection can be introduced into the uterus. The woman will probably wear a hospital gown and if she has not already had a blood test to measure the level of AFP she will have that first. She lies on something like an operating table and an ultrasound scan tells the position of the placenta and the fetus and shows exactly how far the needle should go into the sac in order to get the fluid. The skin of her abdomen is swabbed with antiseptic and a paper sheet with a hole through it where the needle is to be introduced is placed over it. She may be given a local anaesthetic, though this is not always considered necessary, and she should ask for one if she wants it.

A long needle attached to a syringe is then pushed through the skin into the uterus and a little fluid withdrawn. Even in the best centres, in approximately one in 1,000 cases the needle goes into a blood vessel and has to be withdrawn and another attempt made to get clear fluid. Once it is correctly positioned and a quantity of fluid is drawn off into the syringe, about as much as would fill a small coffee cup, some plastic skin may be sprayed on the puncture site and a plaster stuck over it. Many women say that just as they think the test is going to begin they are told it is all over. Even so, it is normal to feel a bit shaky after it.

If you live some way from the hospital it is a good idea to arrange for someone else to drive you home, and then to go straight to bed for a few hours. Do anything which will help you relax. You could listen to music or read an absorbing book. Spend the next week fairly quietly.

The needle puncture made in the amniotic sac is no bigger than the prick made by a rose thorn. It usually seals over automatically once the needle is withdrawn. Occasionally there is some dribbling of fluid and sometimes there is vaginal bleeding. Two per cent of women have some loss of fluid or bleeding.[5]

The risk of miscarriage is low – approximately one per cent – and less in skilled hands. It may be higher for a woman who has had bleeding during pregnancy or who has scars from a previous Caesarean section. Miscarriage after amniocentesis is most likely to occur on the third or fourth day.

The test for Down's syndrome entails growing cells obtained from the amniotic fluid. In between 1 and 5 per cent of all cases the cell culture does not grow. This is discovered in a week to ten days. The woman is then asked to come for another amniocentesis. This can be an ordeal and she may decide that, since an abortion would now take place later still, she is not willing to have repeat amniocentesis.

Ultrasound should always be used with amniocentesis to make quite certain that the needle is placed so that it does not puncture the placenta or harm the baby. In fact the baby usually bounces away like a cork in a beaker of water, but ultrasound increases the safety of the procedure. Damage to the placenta can produce an Rh incompatibility reaction in the circulation of an Rh negative mother if the fetus is Rh positive, leading to rhesus isoimmunization. The mother's blood manufactures antibodies to the baby's blood, destroying some of its red blood cells. The baby becomes anaemic and jaundiced.

You should be able to have a discussion with a genetic counsellor before you decide whether or not to have amniocentesis and, if you go ahead, also to interpret any results about which you want further explanation.

There may also be things you do *not* want to know. One, as we have seen, may be the sex of the baby. You may also decide you do not want to be told about any deviation from the normal which is as yet not understood and where knowledge cannot help you in decision-making. Minor chromosomal abnormalities are quite often detected when analysis is being done for Down's syndrome. Many of us have these slightly abnormal chromosomes and go through our lives without ever discovering it or being hampered by the condition. If parents know that a child lacks a chromosome or possesses an extra one they are likely to wait in apprehension and watch for any sign of abnormal behaviour. Barbara Katz Rothman, in *The Tentative Pregnancy: Prenatal Diagnosis and the Future of Motherhood* (Viking, New York, 1986), makes this point strongly.

Research has shown, for example, that there are more men with an extra Y chromosome in prison than in the general population. The media picked this up and concluded that it was because they must be more aggressive. Subsequent research has indicated that this is not so. (Another theory is that men with an extra Y chromosome are inclined to be rather less intelligent, so they are the ones who get caught!) Imagine knowing that your 2-year-old son had an extra Y chromosome. When he has a tantrum in the supermarket – something a great many 2-year-olds do at one time or another – would you think that this must be because of his extra chromosome and that he's well on the way towards violent crime? Would it make the tasks of parenthood simpler, or more difficult? There are no easy answers to these questions, but certainly acquiring more and more information does not always lead to greater wisdom.

There are some risks and problems with amniocentesis, and for some women these outweigh the benefits. Women often have marked and sometimes regular uterine contractions immediately following amniocentesis. This can be alarming even if you know that it is normal. There are statistical associations between amniocentesis and bleeding in pregnancy, newborn babies who have some difficulties with breathing and babies with orthopaedic handicaps.[6]

In deciding whether or not to have amniocentesis you will want to think through what not having this baby means to you. That cannot be discovered through statistics.

Lynn is 40, with two children, and has decided to have amniocentesis:

> If there's something wrong I'd say I can put up with that. I'd have an abortion. It's for the family as much as for myself. They're here already and they've got feelings. I'd get rid of a handicapped baby for their sake.

Karen, whose partner has a brother with spina bifida, has decided against amniocentesis:

> We've waited so long to have this baby. We've been trying ten years. If I lost it because of amniocentesis I'd never forgive myself, and if it does turn out that the baby is handicapped, well, I expect – I hope – we'd cope. I know couples where a handicapped baby has drawn them very close. I think our love for each other would give us strength.

Gail had a miscarriage after amniocentesis last year. She is 37 and the risks of having a handicapped baby at that age are only slightly greater than those of miscarriage. She says:

> You can't weigh a handicapped baby against a miscarriage. I'd rather have six miscarriages than a handicapped child for life.

Your age, whether or not you conceive easily, your commitment to this pregnancy, your partner's feelings, your acceptance of handicap or the death of a child and your beliefs about and willingness to have abortion all need to be considered. This is not something that doctors can do for you.

Having an abortion

A major problem with amniocentesis is that if the pregnancy is to be terminated it results in a late abortion, after 20 weeks. This can be intensely distressing. Women are sometimes told they should be grateful for the opportunity to get rid of a handicapped baby and that, after all, there is nothing to stop them having another baby very soon afterwards. It may be suggested that losing a child in this way is easier than the loss of a perfect child. That kind of arithmetic has no meaning in terms of personal experience. An amniocentesis abortion is the death of a baby and entails making a painful and often heart-rending choice.

The abortion is often induced with prostaglandins, and pain-killing drugs are readily available. Even so, it is not an experience that any woman would want to go through. One woman described her abortion as 'a hideous mockery of childbirth'. The whole process can take eight hours or more. A woman needs strong emotional support during this time and in the weeks afterwards. At this stage of pregnancy she is likely to lactate once the abortion is over. A tight bra, reduction of fluids and cold compresses against the breasts (ice in a large handkerchief or a packet of frozen peas) will help cope with the discomfort.

Another difficulty with amniocentesis is that the interval between having it done and getting the results is obviously a worrying time. Though some results are available in 24 hours, others take three or four weeks – sometimes longer. A woman often feels she cannot tell other people she is pregnant and make a social reality of it in case abortion lies ahead. Kathy is 39 and has been trying to conceive for eight years. While she was waiting for the test in the genetics department of the hospital she said:

> I haven't told my mother I'm expecting a baby. It seems that everyone knows about it apart from our families. They'd get excited – but I daren't tell them yet until I know the result. We want to avoid any disappointment for them. It's all so unreal – weird. I've been wearing especially floppy clothes so they don't notice. The biggest problem was that when I was staying with them I felt so nauseated in the mornings. I ate breakfast when I didn't feel like it and then tried to go to the bathroom casually so that I could vomit it up. It will be a relief when I can tell them at last – if I ever *can*, that is.

The verdict for which a woman is waiting seems to be a judgement on her ability to bear a healthy baby – even, perhaps, a judgement of her value as a woman. After an amniocentesis abortion she may even feel that this developing life had to be destroyed because she is bad and that she carries death and disease deep in her body. This sense of dreadful personal guilt is made more severe if you are cared for by a nurse who has moral objections to abortion.

Everyone needs a confiding friend who understands what she is going through and accepts the strength of these emotions without trying to argue them away. In fact, a woman has often not told people about her pregnancy and may keep her termination a shameful secret. And even if she has, there may be no one who can understand the storm of conflicting emotions she feels and the guilt and depression which may grip her for months afterwards. Because she has done the 'sensible' thing there may be no recognition of her need to grieve. Friends may say, 'How glad you must be that you found out in time!' Relief and gratitude that the abnormality was detected are the only socially acceptable emotions.

In spite of this, it is usually wise to tell people you are pregnant *before* amniocentesis. Most babies will be fine, and even when both parents are carriers of some defective gene, there is a 3 in 4 chance that it will be good news. And even though it may be difficult to get the emotional support you need if you have to lose this baby, if no one else knew you were pregnant in the first place, you certainly will not receive the help you need.

Amniocentesis is only the first of a whole range of tests and operations that can be done inside the body of the mother. They all raise enormous moral questions about abortion, about the quality of human life, a woman's rights over her own body compared with her responsibility for the fetus, and her personal rights compared with her responsibility to society. In some American states a doctor *must* perform amniocentesis on all women over 35 or be guilty of negligence. It has been suggested that, similarly, a woman over 35 has a duty to have amniocentesis and to abort an imperfect baby.

Though these investigations and operations involve doctors, they are not really medical questions at all. They concern human values and present challenges which we have to meet if we are to accept responsibility for the future. I believe it is wrong merely to be at the receiving end of everything that science makes possible. We have to ask ourselves important questions, and the answers are never easy.

Chorionic villus biopsy

Chorionic villus sampling (CVS) can be done much earlier in pregnancy than amniocentesis – between the sixth and tenth week. A cannula (a fine hollow tube) is introduced through your vagina and cervix, guided by an ultrasound scan, and some chorionic villus tissue is suctioned out. Chorionic villi are projections like miniature ivy roots which stick out from the maternal side of the developing placenta, while it is still at a very early stage, in order to dig themselves into the lining of the uterus so that oxygen and nutritional elements can be carried to the fetus.

Samples of these tissues can be analysed for genetic and metabolic defects, including Down's syndrome and other chromosome abnormalities, thalassaemia, sickle cell anaemia and Tay-Sachs disease.

The waiting time for results is much shorter than with amniocentesis, 24 hours as compared with two to six weeks. The great advantage with this test is that if you decide on termination it can still be done before 12 weeks. At this stage a suction abortion can be performed, whereas in the second trimester a saline or prostaglandin abortion is necessary, which results in what is, to all intents and purposes, a labour.

Though this may seem an ideal method, there remain many questions about CVS which require answers. One concerns the rate of miscarriage following the test, which in some research units has been estimated in the past to be as high as 10 per cent. It is also important to bear in mind that many abnormal fetuses are miscarried spontaneously, so that when termination is done as early as eight weeks, a number of women with fetuses which would have aborted naturally will have had an elective abortion before this can happen.

Other questions concern the rates of pelvic infection, bleeding and leaking of amniotic fluid, and possible developmental abnormalities resulting in low birth-weight in babies who go to term after chorionic villus biopsy. We do not yet know the answers to all these questions, though research is taking place and the outlook for the future is hopeful.

Ultrasound

It took nearly 50 years after the introduction of X-rays for people to realize that they were harmful in pregnancy. Even though warnings about radiation were given in the early twenties, an authority could state in 1935, 'Antenatal work without the routine use of X-rays is no more justifiable than would be the treatment of fractures.'[7] Two years later the Director of the Radiology Department at University College Hospital, London, stated categorically that in the hands of a competent operator there was no danger.[8] In one specialized maternity hospital (Queen Charlotte's) two thirds of pregnant women were having X-rays by 1954, a year when new higher-voltage X-ray equipment was introduced.[9] Two years later Dr Alice Stewart published her findings which revealed that a baby X-rayed in the uterus was twice as likely to die of cancer by the age of 10.[10] It was only then that warnings were heeded and rates of X-rays in pregnancy reduced. Since Marie Curie first worked with radium the dangers of radioactivity had been known, but the knowledge was brushed aside because obstetricians persuaded themselves that the benefits of knowing what was going on inside the uterus outweighed the risks.

Ultrasound was invented during the Second World War and used to detect submarines at sea. By the second half of the fifties obstetric ultrasound was being used in Glasgow. The principle behind it is that sound rays bounce off solid objects. This produces an image on a screen, or a pulsed beam – Doppler ultrasound for fetal heart monitoring. Ultrasound's great advantage is that it does not have the obvious dangers of X-rays and can reveal more of life inside the uterus.

At present there is no evidence that ultrasound is unsafe, but there is a great deal of discussion about its possible delayed and long-term risks. Some people are asking whether, since there was such a long delay in acknowledging the risks of radiation, there may not be hidden dangers in the use of ultrasound in pregnancy.

Until follow-up studies have been done on hundreds of thousands of adults who, when inside the uterus, were exposed to ultrasound, how can we be sure, they say, that we are not playing with fire? And if the majority of women and fetuses show no adverse effects of ultrasound, is it possible that some may be especially vulnerable? [11] Whereas it is agreed that ultrasound can be very useful diagnostically – when it is thought that because the top of the uterus is not as high as it should be at that stage of pregnancy the baby may not be growing well, to locate the placenta when it is lying low, or to reveal a congenital handicap – there is no evidence that its routine use to monitor fetal growth is of benefit.

Today most pregnant women in the Western world are exposed to ultrasound in one form or another and many receive a standard scan – usually at 16 weeks – and at least 20 to 30 minutes of ultrasound in the form of Doppler investigations performed when they go into labour. A good number receive much more than this. Some obstetricians advocate two or three scans routinely in pregnancy, together with fetal heart monitoring in the last weeks. Scans are also used to explore possible abnormalities in the fetus, such as spina bifida and blockages in the gastro-intestinal tract, and may be used in addition to amniocentesis for this purpose.

Having a scan

When you have a scan early in pregnancy you will be asked to drink a lot of water beforehand and come with a full bladder. This clearly distinguishes the bladder and presses the intestines out of the way of the uterus. Your abdomen will first be greased with mineral oil. Then a probe which emits waves of sound too high for the ear to hear is passed over the uterus. This is completely painless for the woman. The sound is translated into dots, each of which is an echo, on a screen like a TV screen. If you want to see it, ask for it to be at an angle where it will be easy for the operator to explain the different parts to you.

At about six weeks the bag of waters can be seen, with the embryo like a small white moon inside. At 16 weeks you can see the heart beating and the position of the placenta, which is often low down in the uterus at this stage. The baby's head is a large white egg-shape. When it twists and turns, the baby is nodding or shaking its head. Sometimes it lifts a hand and starts to suck its thumb. Measurements may be taken from the top of the head to the rump and from one ear across to the other.

With a scan after 24 weeks it may be possible to see the baby's sex, though this depends on how the baby is lying. The genitals of girls often look very plump and large at this stage, so it is easy to mistake a girl for a boy. Sometimes a woman is told her baby's sex incorrectly.

You may be offered a polaroid snap of your baby to take home and stick in the photograph album. The whole process takes about a quarter of an hour.

Diana was thrilled to see her baby: 'It was like looking at a tadpole in a tank. The legs were just little stubbles. I was amazed. I couldn't feel anything but it was moving like anything!'

Frances was so excited when she saw the image of her baby that she shouted out: 'Look! He – she's waving to me!'

Because women often enjoy seeing their babies, some obstetricians believe that a scan enables a mother to 'bond' with her child long before birth. The majority of women in the past have managed to love their babies without this extra technological prodding towards mother love. Intrigued as doctors may be with this response, and happy that they can contribute to it, it is insufficient justification for employing a powerful diagnostic technique in the absence of other reasons for doing so.

The ultrasound scan can provide doctors with a great deal of information about the developing fetus. Between 16 and 24 weeks it should be able to give an accurate dating of pregnancy. After that time it is likely to be wrong.[12] It can show that a fetus is, in all likelihood, normal, can detect some fetal abnormalities without the need for amniocentesis (e.g., spina bifida, anencephaly, and Turner's syndrome – an intersex condition) and can reveal conditions, such as heart defects, tumours and skeletal and urinary tract abnormalities, which would not be disclosed by amniocentesis. In very early pregnancy it shows whether there is tissue inside the amniotic sac and later on whether the baby's heart is beating, so that it is known whether the pregnancy is continuing. It reveals the presence of twins (or more), and the position of the placenta shows up, so that if placenta praevia (the placenta lying over the cervix) is diagnosed a Caesarean birth can be planned in advance. It can diagnose a 'small-for-dates' fetus, though many mistakes are made about this.

But ultrasound also has disadvantages.[13] It often diagnoses conditions, for example a low-lying placenta or placenta praevia, or a malpresentation, which, though present at one phase of pregnancy, have changed by the time labour starts. Results are not always interpreted accurately, so it can suggest that everything is all right when it is not, or that an abnormal condition is present when it is not.[14] After 25 weeks it is very inaccurate in diagnosing fetal maturity.[15] Ultrasound assessment of gestational age is not always as accurate as is often suggested. Sometimes a woman is well aware of when conception must have occurred and she knows that the scan gives an inaccurate date.

Jennie was having her second baby at home. She had one scan at 16 weeks, when she was told she must be 18 weeks. She described her pregnancy as 'perfect'. At 37 weeks a transverse lie was diagnosed – the baby was lying across her uterus – and she was ordered to go into hospital immediately for induction: 'Otherwise the baby may die.' She refused, but said she was 'absolutely terrified'. Two weeks later the baby turned head down. She went into labour spontaneously at what, according to the scan, was 42 weeks and delivered a 7 lb. 6 oz. baby who gave no sign of being 'overdue'. If labour had been induced the baby would have been four to five weeks premature.

In some hospitals ultrasound dating is more reliable than this and obstetricians do not seek to intervene so readily. A controlled trial in Glasgow revealed a 94-per-cent accuracy in identifying babies who were small-for-dates at birth when two scans were done, one before 24 weeks and another between 34 and 36 weeks. Nevertheless, this study failed to show any benefit from the routine use of ultrasound in low-risk pregnancies and the authors concluded that they were 'unable to recommend this schedule as a routine screening method'.[16]

While the short-term safety of diagnostic ultrasound is clear, there remain questions about its long-term safety.[17] It is not yet known whether ultrasound may produce changes in fetal cells which could sometimes lead to cancer much later in life or whether, through changes in DNA and cell structure, it could affect the health of future generations. In mice, ultrasound alters cells after 10 generations of cell division and this persists for up to 100 generations.[18] If there is even an outside chance of this it seems wise to avoid a scan in the first 12 weeks, when the tissues of the fetus are at their most vulnerable stage, unless there are pressing reasons to have one. Finding out after a heavy bleed whether you have miscarried or are about to miscarry might be one of these for some women. (Others prefer to wait and see.)

The use made of information gained from ultrasound, and how this affects the rest of the pregnancy and the way labour is managed, is an issue discussed in medical journals but not much talked about by the general public or from the woman's point of view. Yet that is an important aspect of ultrasound policy. If it is unlikely to alter care, it is pointless. If the response to the information is anxiety on the part of the doctor or the mother – or both – which cannot be canalized into constructive action, ultrasound can have a negative effect on the rest of the pregnancy. If it leads to women being admitted to hospital unnecessarily or having unnecessary inductions or Caesarean sections, the effect is also negative.

Though in Britain the Royal College of Obstetricians and Gynaecologists has accepted a policy of routine scanning at 16 weeks, there is no evidence that ultrasound is of any benefit when used routinely. This is recognized by the American College of Obstetricians and Gynecologists, which has issued a statement that 'no well-controlled study has yet proved that routine scanning of all prenatal patients will improve the outcome of pregnancy' [19] and recommends that 'at present, only indicated diagnostic studies should be ordered'.

If you are advised to have ultrasound there are some questions you may want to ask:[20]

What information is it expected to provide?
Is this important?
If so, why?
How accurate will it be at this stage of pregnancy?
How will it affect my pregnancy if I do not have a scan?
Will enough be learned to justify exposing the baby to the possible risk of ultrasound?

You may want to ensure that the results of a scan will be given to you on the spot, and that often happens only if a doctor is present. The radiographer is normally expected to report to your obstetrician.

You may also want to know if a record of the number of scans you have, intensity of exposure and the time exposed to ultrasound is kept. Unless records like this are kept it is impossible to know if there are any long-term effects.

You may wish to have an assurance that your partner will be able to be with you. This not only reduces any anxiety, but can make it an exciting shared experience.

At this stage it might be useful to get out your notebook and, perhaps in discussion with your partner or a friend, jot down your main conclusions. Decide which questions you would want to ask if ultrasound was advised by your obstetrician and make a note of these.

Doppler ultrasound

Ultrasound is also used to monitor the fetal heart-beat, both prenatally and in labour, either in the form of a transducer pressed over the site of the baby's heart from outside the mother's abdomen and attached to her by a tight belt, or as a sonic aid, about the size of a small tape recorder, used intermittently. The other kind of continuous monitoring is done electronically by means of an electrode attached to a screw or clip which is introduced through the mother's cervix and stuck into the baby's scalp. This kind does not employ ultrasound.

When ultrasound is used for fetal heart monitoring it often gives information which is misinterpreted, so producing false positives and false negatives.[21] Women are required to lie down when a trace is being recorded. This can cause compression of the large blood vessels in the lower part of the mother's body, reduced blood flow to the baby, and hence heart-rate abnormalities. It is also often extremely uncomfortable for her to stay in one position like this in order to get a clear print-out, and she feels constricted and inhibited.

The immediate effect of ultrasound on the baby is rarely discussed, but a pregnant woman who is being monitored usually notices that the fetus responds by jumping around. In fact, in late pregnancy this is employed as a test of fetal vitality and the baby's movements often feel quite wild. As with a dog-whistle, our ears cannot pick up the sound waves, but for the baby it may be as shrill and powerful as the noise of a police siren. The conditions in which most women are examined often prove stressful enough to make the baby move vigorously. One study reported acceleration of the fetal heart rate when doctors came to the woman's bedside.[22]

Even in high-risk pregnancies fetal heart recording does not mean that more babies' lives are saved. In studies of routine heart monitoring more babies die in the groups having it than in the control groups which do not have it.[23] Certainly the use of ultrasound in pregnancy, in the words of the US Department of Health and Human Services, 'should be limited to situations in which there is an accepted medical reason for the procedure . . . There is not enough evidence that routine screening benefits either the mother or the fetus.'

So, with Doppler monitoring, as with the ultrasound scan, it would seem sensible to keep levels as low as possible and only agree to be monitored if their are clinical signs that all may not be well.

Testing for herpes

Genital herpes can cause miscarriage and premature birth, and blindness and sometimes death in the newborn baby. This tends to be an infection of the middle and upper-middle classes, not of lower socio-economic groups. If a woman has had active herpes in pregnancy a culture is usually taken six weeks before the baby is due and then again two weeks before to check that the disease has cleared. Some obstetricians, however, believe the right point at which to test is once labour has started, and recommend that all women should have this done. Vaginal delivery is usually considered safe if no lesions have appeared in the last eight days. When a culture is positive, however, or there are lesions, a Caesarean birth is advised.[24]

If a baby is to be born vaginally, the important fact is not whether you have had herpes, but the condition of your vagina *when labour starts*, and this especially if you have developed herpes for the first time (primary herpes) during this pregnancy. A woman who has had herpes in the past transmits antibodies through the placenta to the baby, who is very unlikely to get the infection. Even if there is a recurrence of herpes during pregnancy there is only a 2- to 3-per-cent chance that the baby will be affected, compared with a 50-per-cent chance if she gets herpes for the first time during pregnancy and has it at the time of birth. That is the real problem: getting an initial attack of herpes when pregnant and having the virus in your genital tract at the time of birth.

Many unnecessary Caesarean sections have been performed because women have had a *recurrence* of herpes, when the babies would very likely have already produced antibodies to the virus. However, if you plan to have a vaginal delivery, and there is any chance of herpes being present, you should aim for birth with as little intervention as possible, because a baby can acquire the virus via a puncture site of an electrode clip in the scalp or breaks in the skin made by forceps.[25]

Chemotherapy is given to any baby who may have been exposed to an active lesion, but is only effective before symptoms are visible. Herpes can also be transmitted after birth from nurses' hands. This is one reason why you may emphasize that you do not want your baby to go to a hospital nursery but to stay by your side all the time.

Hormone tests or kick charts?

Because the placenta is the baby's life-line, obstetricians want to find more effective ways of monitoring its function. One test involves measuring the level of oestriol, an oestrogen hormone in the mother's urine which is produced jointly by the baby's liver and the placenta. As the baby grows, more oestriol is excreted. Since there are usually large fluctuations in the production of oestriol at different times of the day, specimens must be taken over a period of 24 hours. It is common practice to admit women to hospital while the urine is collected, though there is really no reason why a woman should not be able to do it herself if she follows instructions carefully.

As a test, however, urinary oestriol is not very reliable in predicting the state of the fetus. For example, a kidney infection can reduce it. In a twin pregnancy it may be lower than anticipated, too. Even taking drugs such as aspirin or ampicillin can affect the oestriol level. It is probably unwise to agree to induction of labour or a Caesarean section merely on the evidence of a low oestriol level.

Other tests are available and are preferred by some obstetricians. These measure oestradiol in blood and human placental lactogen (HPL), a hormone produced by the placenta itself. Though they are often more accurate, they entail frequent blood tests.

Keeping a daily record of fetal movements is more reliable in assessing fetal well-being than chemical tests.[26]

If the placenta is not functioning well to provide oxygen and nourishment for the baby, the number and strength of fetal movements decreases. When a baby dies it stops moving altogether at least 12 hours beforehand. Some babies who are perfectly all right, however, have long periods when there are no obvious movements. Perhaps they are just sleeping.

In one research project, of 78 women who felt no movement at all for 12 hours or longer, 66 gave birth to babies in good condition one to ten weeks later. Obstetricians decided that the other 12 babies were safer out than in and delivered them. Ten of these were in peak condition at birth and only two were at all stressed.[27]

Obstetricians may prefer chemical hormone tests because they do not really trust women to keep records. Some suspect they will cheat, or may not realize when their babies move or may forget to keep the charts. It is difficult for some doctors to hand over that kind of power to women.

Even though mothers themselves are the best judges of their babies' vitality, and though fetal movement records kept by them are more reliable than the other tests, kick charts can cause great anxiety if they are kept only for the purpose of checking whether the baby is still alive. It seems best to limit their use to the very end of pregnancy and only for a part of each day, as a way of getting in touch with the baby and learning its sleeping and waking times and rhythms of activity and rest. Most babies move at least 10 times in a 12-hour period – some much more – but a woman does not notice many of these movements, either because they are slight, or because she is preoccupied and busy doing other things. If you have a good deal of amniotic fluid it may not be easy to detect separate movements. If you do not have very much you may feel that the baby is moving all the time. If you are having twins it will probably feel like a basketful of wriggling puppies.

Some women really enjoy keeping movement charts. Carol said:

> They told me one week I had put on far too much weight and I almost starved myself the next week. Then they told me I had lost weight and they were worried about that. I'd been keeping a kick chart anyway, for fun. It was good to be *doing* something and when the doctor said, 'You haven't put on any weight' to be able to say, 'Well the baby is kicking a lot. Here is my kick chart.'

Other women dislike movement charts. Jane said:

> I never could work out what was a movement and what wasn't, and was always wondering whether I should count it. I got very fraught.

Keeping a movement chart

If you would like to make your own movement chart you will need some squared paper. At the top left of your page write the time you are going to start counting movements, selecting a time when your baby is most active. This is often in the evening. But you may prefer to do it in the morning if you tend to worry at night. Divide the squares by half hours down the page. Across the top of the page write the days of the week and the date. It may look like this:

Time			Aug. 1/7								Aug. 8/14				
	M	Tu	W	Th	F	Sat	Sun	M	Tu	W	Th	F	Sat	Sun
9.30														
10.00														
10.30														
11.00														

and so on

Each day you are going to count up to the tenth movement, always starting at the same time. Then block in the square which covers the half-hour when you felt the tenth kick. You should feel that kick at about the same time each day, give or take half an hour or so, though the baby may become very quiet in the 12 hours just before you start labour. If you do not notice 10 movements in 12 hours, make a note of the number of movements you felt in that time and let your doctor know. Do this if you cannot as a rule feel 10 kicks in 12 hours and also if, having previously felt more, you notice now that movements are much less. The obstetrician will probably suggest listening to the fetal heart, perhaps using Doppler ultrasound. The likelihood is that you will be assured all is well.

The detection of pathology is an important part of an obstetrician's task. But it should not be the only one. What amounts to the constant ringing of alarm bells in pregnancy can sometimes produce the very abnormalities which obstetricians are trying to avoid.

Even the advice that is given to a woman in pregnancy can have such an effect. If you are worried about the terrible damage you could do to your baby by smoking or drinking alcohol, it could be that you turn to these things for comfort because you feel so miserable. If you are sick with worry that the baby is not growing properly and you are not putting on enough weight, it may be that the tension this produces can affect your metabolism and the baby's nutrition in the uterus so as to bring about the condition you are trying to avoid. If you live each day with the threat of raised blood pressure and its dreadful consequences hanging over you, this can actually cause your blood pressure to go up.

Recognition of deviations from the norm is valuable. But an even more important element in the care a pregnant woman receives ought to be support for everything that is going *right*. Many obstetricians have no idea of how to do this. They are expert at tracking down things that might go wrong, but completely at a loss as to how to preserve and enhance the normal.

This is where a woman's confidence and determination to reclaim her body in pregnancy is vital, and the basis for a positive experience of childbirth.

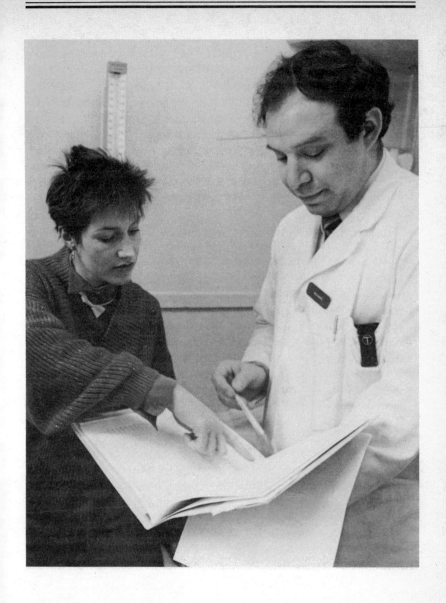

*Being Positive
and Taking Action*

10

SAYING WHAT YOU WANT

A pregnant woman needs special skills to negotiate the kind of care that she believes is right for her, sometimes with doctors who are firmly convinced that they know better. Obstacles may be put in her way. Information may be hard to obtain. Sometimes she may feel she is beating her head against a brick wall. To cope with this she needs to be quietly, firmly, persistently and imperturbably *assertive.*

To be assertive is to make a clear statement about what you think and want, and set limits on what other people do to you. You appear confident (even if you don't feel it inside) and can act decisively. Self-confidence grows out of the practice of assertion.

This is quite different from being aggressive. An aggressor accuses and attacks other people, intent on destroying the enemy. Aggression creates adversaries and each encounter is like a battle between opposing armies, after which you each chalk up the results: win or lose.

It is incredibly difficult to start suddenly being assertive with doctors if you are not already accustomed to speaking out and saying what you want. Yet it is especially important to do this in pregnancy and childbirth, if only because otherwise they cannot know what you really want. They may make assumptions about the kind of birth and the drugs you are going to have and the way you want your baby cared for, because of a set of expectations they have acquired from medical school, or simply because this is how they have always treated patients in the past. Many women grumble about what happened in the doctor's surgery or have a quiet weep afterwards, but do not make their dissatisfaction clear to the doctor. He (for it usually is a he) can hardly be blamed for not picking up clues to what the woman wanted, since they were so muted and vague that he could ignore them, or swamp them with his personal style of patient management – whether this was one of fatherly protection, 'all pals together', or blind-you-with-science space-age obstetrics – so that the woman went away feeling diminished, almost as if she did not exist as a person any more.

If you get on well with your doctor you may never have wanted to be assertive, and may question the need for it. To examine what is going on between you may even seem unfriendly and can make you feel very uncomfortable. But how this relationship works is not just a matter of two individuals liking each other, but of how behaviour between doctors and patients is *socially* organized.

The relationship between a patient and a doctor is one of unequal power, however kind and friendly the doctor. This is so whether the patient is male or female, but it is especially marked when the doctor is male and the patient a pregnant woman who is anxious to do the best for her baby – particularly if it is her first child.

In Western culture professionals have largely taken over the power of the priesthood. They control the dangerous passages through crises in our lives. They bring their special and often costly expertise both to judge us and to mediate on our behalf with destiny. This occurs in a particularly dramatic way, and one depicted vividly by the media, with heart surgeons, but it also happens, for example, with lawyers, teachers and professors, psychiatrists – and gynaecologists and obstetricians. The esoteric knowledge of the professional can be exploited to exert power over a lay person.

The relationship between a woman patient and her doctor is especially lop-sided because women are dependent on doctors for basic control of their reproductive functions: getting and not getting pregnant, staying or not staying pregnant, and childbirth itself.[1] Even a perfectly healthy woman is dependent on them for overseeing her body's normal functions. Gynaecologists and obstetricians have become the representatives of women's bodies, with specialist and esoteric information to which women themselves are not supposed to have access. The women's health movement has started to break down these barriers of knowledge, but there are still many women who prefer to 'trust' the doctor and to leave all important decisions about their bodies to him.

When a woman and her doctor both accept this pattern their relationship tends to be friction-free. When either tries to shift the balance towards equality confusion may result. An obstetrician was talking to me about his feelings of frustration when asking women to make choices between alternatives. Over and over again they would say, 'I leave it to you, Doctor.'

Most obstetricians are as much part of the system, and trapped in it, as their women patients. They sometimes take their superior knowledge so much for granted, and the kind of information they have about patients as so much more valid, that medical records appear to have more reality than anything their patients can say about themselves. Ann Oakley reports part of an interview between an obstetrician and his patient in a large, prestigious London teaching hospital:[2]

DOCTOR [*reading case notes*]: Ah, I see you've got a boy and a girl.
PATIENT: No, two girls.
DOCTOR: Really, are you sure? I thought it said . . . [*checks in case notes*] Oh no, you are quite right, two girls.

It can be very difficult to start being assertive in medical encounters. It is as if we are pre-programmed to surrender power, to abrogate choice and trust the authority of experts. Taking positive action in our relationships with doctors means that we need to accept what can be frightening responsibility for the outcome of choices we make. It also entails acknowledgement of the help and guidance doctors can give us to get the information we want and to weigh up the pros and cons of alternative courses of action.

One problem in becoming assertive is that there may be no reward for it. It is unlikely that anyone will say 'Well done!' and you may be left feeling that you have committed a grave social error. A doctor who does not usually deal with assertive women may be confused and on the defensive. You will probably notice his discomfort and may be concerned about it. But it is vital to prevent yourself slipping into a passive mode. Women are brought up to care for others and to be nurturing. We are taught to be aware of their emotions, to be warm and comforting, and especially to make men feel good about themselves. We smile. We soothe. We admire. There are many good things about this, if men were able to behave in the same way. But they usually do not. They are the executives. They direct and manage. They are 'too busy' with important matters to concern themselves with emotions. Obviously not all men are like this. But most are trained in this style from boyhood. They are taught to dominate, to beat the other guy and, above all, to be strong.

So feeling sorry for the doctor is a danger signal. Only one step from there and a woman starts to placate, reassure, apologize and retract whatever she said she wanted. And like the Cheshire cat in *Alice in Wonderland*, in the end only her smile remains. You do not have to make your doctor feel comfortable at the expense of your own discomfort. Though it is important that you recognize and understand them, you are not responsible for his emotions. Let him know what kind of help and support you need. When he gives it, say that you appreciate it. If you are not getting it, say how you feel and what you want with greater clarity. If he seems unable to give it, change your doctor. Contact your local Family Practitioner Committee (which will be in the phone book) and ask for the names of G Ps on the obstetric list. If you cannot find a doctor who seems right for you but there are independent midwives, go straight to a midwife. In Britain you are not legally obliged to be attended by a doctor. The Association of Radical Midwives or the Independent Midwives' Association may be able to give you some names. The Senior Nursing Officer for Community Midwifery will also be able to help you. A trained midwife is qualified to give complete care before and after the baby comes, and during a normal birth, without the help of a doctor. She calls in a doctor when and if necessary. Childbirth organizations can almost invariably help you find another doctor or a midwife too. There is a list of these organizations on p. 311.

It takes pluck to move out from the carefully created image of a woman who always understands and can put herself in another person's place and sympathize, to the different image of a decisive, go-getting woman who refuses to take no for an answer, who can state her case with verve, stand her ground and employ a planned strategy to achieve what is important to her. As women, we have been conditioned not to like ourselves that way. But when you are having a baby it is really worth it.

Before you can take control of your pregnancy effectively you need to discover what your rights are. These are often not clearly defined in law, though the childbirth organizations should be able to help you. But you do need to know, for example, that it is legal to have a baby at home, though in some parts of North America it may be illegal to have a midwife attend you. In Britain, however, you *must* call a midwife. And if you have your baby in hospital it may be useful to know, for example, that you can insist on not having your baby separated from you. The baby belongs to you, not to the hospital.

There is always a price to pay for not being assertive, and it helps to look at this, in terms both of feelings at the time and of later consequences. Here is what one woman said:

> In my first labour my midwife told me I needed pethidine [an analgesic drug related to morphine]. I didn't want it so I said so. She said, 'You don't realize how painful it's going to get. You can cope now but I shall be scraping you off the walls in two hours' time if you don't have it now.' So I let her give me a shot. I think she may have given me another when I was too drowsy to resist at all. When the baby was born I was so doped that I didn't even remember I wanted to hold her immediately and put her to the breast. I let them put her in a plastic box and wheel her off to the nursery. I

bitterly regretted it afterwards. I feel I cheated her out of something that was her birthright.

When you are pregnant there are many blocks in the way of being assertive. You may be taken by surprise by a decision – to induce labour, for example – and not have considered what you want. Or before you can come to any decision you may need some information which is difficult to obtain, so are left floundering while an obstetrician puts pressure on you to have a Caesarean section because your baby is breech, for example, and justifies this with a blanket statement that 'it is safer for the baby'. If you don't know what questions to ask, you may feel that you will look silly if you attempt to be assertive, especially if it is your first baby. Suppose, for example, that having read about the advantages of squatting and semi-squatting positions for delivery, you ask if you can give birth on the floor in an upright position, but your doctor says that the baby will fall on the floor and may suffer brain damage. Unless you realize that a woman spontaneously bends her knees and crouches down from the standing position as she presses the baby out, and that, with any delivery, someone should be there with hands waiting to cradle the baby's head if necessary, you may feel that you will look foolish in continuing to ask for this.

Women are often vulnerable because they are concerned about the effects of their decisions on the baby. That is why emotional blackmail by those who threaten that if you do not obey you can harm the baby is so effective. Get in touch with birth and other consumer organizations which can help you, seek another professional opinion if necessary, and ask whether there have been controlled clinical trials to produce reliable evidence. Then, either stand your ground and refuse the intervention, or, if you can discover a more enlightened obstetrician or midwife, change your care-giver.

Arguing is rarely the most effective way of being assertive. *You do not have to produce arguments at all.* It is enough to say: 'No, thank you' . . . 'I have decided against it' . . . 'I need time to think about that' . . . 'I want to discuss it with X before I make up my mind' . . . 'I do not give my consent to this' . . . or simply 'Please, stop doing that.' If you are asked why, you can repeat your statement, add one of the other statements in this list, or say how you feel. Other people may not agree with you, but they must acknowledge the validity of your feelings.

There is great value in repetition. It has been called the 'technique of the cracked record'. When you use repetition quietly but firmly, you cannot be driven off-course.

Maggie, for example, has just become pregnant and is choosing her obstetrician. She talked to other women who went to Dr Z and learnt that he insisted on electronic fetal monitoring for each one. Maggie is keen to have an active birth and move around in labour. She knows that continuous electronic fetal monitoring usually restricts movement. She wants to know how many of Dr Z's patients have electronic fetal monitoring.

MAGGIE: Would you tell me the proportion of women you care for who have continuous electronic fetal monitoring? Is it routine for everyone?

DOCTOR: Nothing is routine in my practice, young lady.

MAGGIE: What is the proportion of women who have electronic fetal monitoring?

DOCTOR: It is used when there is a medical indication.

MAGGIE: I see. What proportion of your patients have it?

DOCTOR: You've been reading *books*!

MAGGIE [*smiling*]: Yes! And I'd like to know how many of the women you care for actually have continuous electronic fetal monitoring.

DOCTOR [*wagging a finger at her*]: You can't learn everything from books, you know.

MAGGIE: I'm sure I can't. That's why I'd like to hear what proportion of women receive it.

DOCTOR: I don't have the figures right here.

MAGGIE: I'd appreciate those figures before I make another appointment with you. But could you make an informed guess now?

DOCTOR: Well, I have many high risk patients with very precious babies. I'd say 85 per cent of my patients benefit from monitoring.

MAGGIE: Thank you, Doctor.

The danger point occurred when the doctor accused her of reading books. Maggie could have turned aggressive, retreated shamefacedly into passivity or started arguing. She did not. She kept cool, agreed with a smile that books cannot teach you everything and firmly and politely repeated her request. She now knows that at least 85 per cent of Dr Z's patients have continuous electronic fetal monitoring – and achieved what she wished in the interview.

One difficult thing to deal with is personal criticism. We all have our vulnerable areas. Here again, ideas about what it is to be a woman play a large part. An accusation that you are insensitive, or criticism of the way you care for your children, your personal appearance or your relationship with your partner may hurt, or at least take the wind out of your sails!

Holly found it difficult to be assertive with her mother, who longed to be needed and involved in every aspect of Holly's pregnancy and birth. She felt there was a risk of her mother taking over the whole experience from her. Her mother worried about her and still thought of her as a little girl who would never be able to look after a baby. Holly decided to be assertive:

> MOTHER: I don't want to interfere, dear, but I hope you're not insisting on Bob watching the birth.
> HOLLY: Yes, Mother. He's looking forward to it. We're reading books together and he's coming to classes with me.
> MOTHER: I think you're laying up trouble for your marriage. Your father and I have been talking about it.
> HOLLY: Bob feels as strongly as I do that he wants to be there.
> MOTHER: You don't understand what birth is like. It's bloody and messy and very, very painful.
> HOLLY: No, I agree that I don't really know what it's like. I'm sorry that it was so awful for you, Mother, and I know things may be different from how we plan them. We want to be flexible to do whatever we feel is right at the time. But from where we are now, we want to share this experience.
> MOTHER: He'll never want to make love to you again!
> HOLLY: Bob likes to feel the baby kicking inside me. We feel very close, Mother. Much closer than before. And we've made up our minds that this is an important part of the way we express our love for each other. I realize that it wouldn't have suited you and Dad, but Bob and I agree that this is how we want it.

Ultimately, assertiveness comes from feeling good about yourself and from a sense of self-worth. Manoeuvres designed to express what you do not feel usually seem artificial and strained. But self-confidence can grow from taking the first steps towards being positive and practising self-assertion.

11

BIRTH PLANS

A birth plan is a concise written statement of your wishes for childbirth and the days following birth, worked out beforehand in consultation with your midwife or doctor. One copy is filed with your records or clipped to your partogram (graphic labour record), the other you keep yourself. It outlines the kind of care you would like and your general approach to the birth experience. It is not a legal document and has no formal binding power, but it gives an opportunity for everyone to understand the things which are most important to you. It is especially vital to have one if you do not know in advance who will be caring for you in labour, and may encounter complete strangers. A birth plan should also take into account the care you would like if labour is not straightforward or if there are deviations from the normal – if you have a Caesarean section, for example, or if the baby goes to the special-care nursery.

There are those who dismiss birth plans as 'shopping lists' that bear no relation to what actually happens in labour, and say that compiling them gives women false expectations and triggers defensive attitudes, and sometimes outright hostility, in doctors and midwives. This is often true. It happens because we don't yet know how to use birth plans in the most effective way, and there are many misconceptions about what a plan can do and how it should be drawn up.

Let us look first at the arguments against birth plans – arguments which any woman may encounter if she raises the question of how she would like her birth to be:

'Don't plan ahead. Keep an open mind. Wait and see. Then you won't be disappointed.' Superficially praiseworthy – and even caring – this kind of advice is usually unhelpful. Birth is a major life event, and for many of us it is also a crisis – even though one we welcome. It involves often overwhelming emotions, and, especially in the late first stage, a sense of being a little boat lost in a storm at sea and out of sight of land, caught in cross-currents, with waves dashing upon waves. Any woman who avoids thinking through in advance how she may feel, what she may want to do and how she wants to be treated as she goes through this momentous experience, is likely to be coerced and swept along by *other* people's assumptions about what is appropriate, who then make decisions *for* her. Many women who have suffered a labour like that, even one which was straightforward and ostensibly easy, look back on it as an ordeal, not only because of pain, but because they felt trapped, confused and totally out of control – a phrase which occurs again and again in women's birth accounts.

The process of constructing a birth plan – seeking the information on which to base your plan, considering the advantages and disadvantages of different courses of action, discussing ideas with a sympathetic midwife or doctor – can be an important means of facing up to the reality of birth as a major life event and growing in self-confidence.

Another argument often used against birth plans is that it sets a woman up to feel afterwards that she has failed. This is often stated categorically, though there has been no research comparing the birth experiences and post-partum emotional states of women with birth plans and those without. This viewpoint derives from an erroneous idea of what a birth plan is. For it should not be a blueprint of how labour 'ought' to be or how you 'should' behave. It is not a description of how a perfect birth would be.

Nor is a birth plan a list of prohibitions to hand to your doctor. It is much more a way of saying 'if such-and-such occurs, then I should like . . .' A birth plan is rather like a plan for a walking or cycling trip – you find out beforehand where you are going and, since the journey can be modified depending how you feel at the time, get information about alternative routes and consider what action can be taken if the going is tough. It follows that a birth plan needs to be constructed bearing in mind that you may make a different decision in labour from the one you envisaged yourself making during pregnancy. You may have thought you would want to eat, for example, and not be able to face food. You may not have wanted an epidural, but find that severe pain leads you to make the decision to have one.

This is not a matter of success or failure, but of an active process of preparation in which you are able to share decision-making about your body and retain your autonomy as a human being. One of the problems with some kinds of birth education in the past is that they either taught women a brave independence which tended to ignore – and sometimes cut off the labouring woman from – the help and support a skilled midwife could give, or it instructed women in how to adapt gracefully and gratefully to whatever was done to them, on the grounds that the doctor always knows best. That this is changing now, and that women and midwives are learning how to work together constructively, is at least partly attributable to the new emphasis on prenatal discussion which explores values important to the pregnant woman and acknowledges her right to accept responsibility for an experience in which she is an active birth-giver rather than a passive patient.

Another accusation that may be levelled against a woman who wishes to make birth plans is that she is thinking only of herself and her own emotional satisfaction, and is ignoring the baby. Obstetricians often consider themselves guardians of the fetus and believe the woman incapable, by reason of her sex, of making rational decisions and, because of a heightened emotional state in pregnancy, prone to flout safety. One obstetrician, Harold Francis, has pronounced that pregnant women should never be allowed to make or even to share in any decisions about their care because they are 'not only emotionally unstable, they are intensely egocentric . . . In this egocentric state, encouragement to participate can result in a fierce demand to dictate.'[1] Here again, there is no research which demonstrates that obstetricians are more concerned about babies than the babies' mothers.

The implication is that the mother's and the baby's needs are quite separate and that the woman's physical and emotional well-being has nothing to do with the baby's welfare. Enough is understood now about the feto-maternal circulation to know that the fear which produces over-breathing and hyperventilation can reduce the fetal oxygen supply, and that an excess of catecholamines (hormones which are over-produced in situations of acute or continuing stress) can result in prolonged labour and, because they pass through the placenta into the baby's bloodstream, may also lead to a reduction in the baby's oxygen supply.[2] A woman in labour is not merely a contracting uterus, as she tends to be described in some obstetric textbooks. Nor is the baby only 'the passenger'. The mother and child are in partnership.

Another argument against birth plans is that they destroy, or do not permit to develop, a relationship between doctor and patient which is based on trust. (This means that the patient trusts her doctor – not, as far as I can gather, the other way round.) 'Trust,' as Michael Klein rightly points out, 'can't be mandated by contract.'[3] It is true that you need to have a good working relationship with whoever is caring for you. This cannot be guaranteed by rules and regulations, whether they are laid down by the doctor or by you. But is it really a matter of 'trusting' the doctor, or rather of the two achieving a partnership in which there is mutual respect? A birth plan can be one expression of a good working relationship between equal partners, each knowing what the task entails, bringing their own skills, recognizing those which the other person has, and each knowing their limits. This is quite different from a woman having unquestioning trust in her doctor, and from the mystique which blankets a relationship in which the doctor assumes an almost priest-like role.

Because care-givers are often opposed to the very idea of birth plans, and extremely anxious about them, you may find you need to reassure them about why you want to make one. You can explain that you are flexible, will accept intervention if you consider it necessary, and are glad to have advice (even if your conclusions may be different from those your doctor would come to).

Of course there will be occasions when a woman will make a decision which the obstetrician or midwife considers wrong, or one which later proves to be wrong: she elects to have an epidural and has an otherwise unnecessary forceps delivery; or she decides on home birth and has to be transferred to hospital during labour; she refuses the offer of episiotomy and has a third-degree tear; or she declines continuous electronic fetal monitoring – and, tragically, the baby dies. It is a very common psychological response in such situations to blame someone else. The woman blames her care-givers. The obstetrician blames the woman – and often the midwife, too.

When a woman accepts responsibility for a decision, she also accepts responsibility for the outcome of that decision, and it cannot be off-loaded on to the obstetrician. This is one reason why the making of birth plans needs careful discussion about the degree of responsibility that is sought and the way in which it is to be shared between the woman giving birth and those helping her. It also means that she must have honest information, in terms she can understand.

In practice many women find that they are subjected to crude emotional blackmail. A woman is threatened, for example, that if she does not 'toe the line' and deliver in hospital, or agree to induction because she has reached 42 weeks, she is risking the baby's life. (Home birth and induction are both subjects of a good deal of obstetric bullying.) It is for the woman to consider the pros and cons of this in the light of her own beliefs and values. Ultimately it is not a medical but a moral decision. No one else has the right to take that responsibility from her if she makes the decision to accept it.

So the main issue concerning birth plans is that of responsibility and control. Are doctors willing to return control of women's bodies in childbirth? Are women confident enough to accept responsibility for our own bodies and for our babies?

In Britain hospitals are increasingly designing their own, formal birth plans and asking women to state their preferences in advance. In some ways this is a sign of progress in communication, and a genuine effort to create a better environment for birth. But many hospital birth plans tend to ignore or to trivialize these fundamental questions of responsibility and control. They provide, instead, a framework within which selected choices are invited: 'Do you want to wear your own nightie or a hospital gown? Yes or no?' Or they request approval for a nowadays customary procedure: 'Do you want to hold your baby immediately after birth? Please tick the appropriate box.' Birth plans can be employed merely as a facade for the insidious institutional control of the whole birth process.

The concept of consumer choice is useful for women having babies when it makes us think about our priorities and compare what we want with the services offered. But it can be misleading when it suggests that we have choice when there is really none but the most trivial, or when it gives an entirely false impression of the degree of courage and initiative women have to find if, making their own informed decisions, they insist on choosing something which is not already on the set 'menu' presented by the medical system.

As hospitals come to treat childbearing women as 'consumers', there is danger that the ethics, the management style and even the advertising techniques of competitive business are introduced, and birth plans run the risk of being used as a softening-up treatment and a sweetener to obtain what the drug companies call 'patient cooperation', conditioning women to put their trust in the professionals who control the birth place.

The creation of a birth plan can be an educational process for all concerned. It stimulates dialogue with those caring for you and prepares the way for a working partnership in which they understand your priorities and are aware of your hopes and fears. It brings out into the open exactly what you expect of your birth companion, whether that is your partner or someone else of your choice, and helps you to talk together about what you want and expect of each other. And it enables you to focus on your role in birth in a positive way, triggering an active search for more information and deeper understanding of the whole experience of birth.

When you reach the end of this book you will have a lot of ideas on which to base your own birth plan. But even at this point you can begin to think about the more general issues, such as 'Where do I want to give birth?', 'Who do I want to attend me?' and 'Who else would I like to be with me to share the experience?'

Your birth companion

The father of your baby may be your best birth companion. A woman often says that it was his hands she sought, his strength on which she relied, and even that she does not know how she could have gone through it without him. For many couples it is a peak experience in their lives, and one they would not have missed sharing together for the world. Yet sometimes another woman best fills that role, and the mother should have freedom to choose who she has with her in labour, and whether that is just one person or several.

Discuss everything in your plan with whoever is going to be your birth companion. This person needs to understand not only what you want but the *way you think* about these subjects, so that you can relax, sure that if necessary he or she will say, 'Hold on! Can you ask her about this first?', or 'I think she wanted to manage without that,' or 'I know she'd like you to help her . . .'

There have been various studies which show the importance of a birth companion, someone concerned exclusively with supporting the woman in labour, and this not only because of the psychological benefits but also because it affects physiological function, helps the birth process unfold more naturally, leads to less intervention, and increases the physical well-being of both mother and baby.[4] In Latin American countries fathers are rarely present, so it was decided to investigate the effect of having a woman companion, not specially trained, to befriend each woman labouring in a Guatemalan hospital. One interesting aspect of this research is that the women did not know their companions beforehand. Even so, their friendship had a remarkable effect. Labours were much shorter; there were twice as many obstetric interventions (including oxytocin augmentation of uterine action and Caesarean birth) in the labours of mothers who had no companion, and twice as many complications during labour (including meconium staining and fetal distress). When she had a companion the mother responded more positively to the sight of her newborn baby and cuddled and talked to it more in the first hour after birth. Fewer babies needed to be brought back into hospital in the first six months of life.

So there is a strong case to be made for having a companion with you in labour, even if this is not the father of the baby; and if he does not seem to be the right person to give you the best emotional support, or is unable to be with you, you may choose to have someone else, or another woman companion as well. Some women feel support is best when they have a group of people to whom they feel close, but unless you are very sure that this is what you want, it is probably wise to limit the number of people around you, if only because you need to focus on your own experience, not theirs, and should not feel that you are having to put on a performance for them.

Your other children

In traditional cultures children are often present during birth. A Zulu chief explained to me that it is an important part of children's education about the precious nature of life to witness both birth and death. When I was doing anthropological research in Jamaica I saw children running in and out of the room during labour or curling up in bed beside their mother. In Mexico and other parts of Latin America the other women present at the birth, helping and encouraging, often have their own children with them.[5]

In the same way that children see preparation of food and cooking going on around them, and are aware of the skills and rhythms of household tasks, so in many Third World cultures they see preparation for birth and the heavy work of labour, and become aware of the skills and rhythms in the group of women attending a birth. This probably results in a more realistic and informed attitude to birth-giving than that of many young women and men who grow up knowing nothing about birth except what they have read in books and magazines or seen in the occasional film.

Though there has been little systematic study and follow-up of the presence of children at birth, such evidence that does exist suggests that this is usually a positive experience for children.[6]

Robbie had seven people with her for Jason's birth: her husband Robert, two midwives, a male friend who took photographs, the godfather-to-be, another woman friend and her 3-year-old daughter, and Robbie's own 4-year-old, Peyton. She had had a previous Caesarean section for 'failure to progress' and was determined to give birth vaginally at home if possible. In Britain no obstetrician would have assumed that she needed a Caesarean the second time round, but she was in the United States where most obstetricians take it for granted that 'once a Caesarean, always a

Caesarean'. So if she wanted an autonomous birth her only option was to labour at home and hope that she did not need to go into hospital.

The labour lasted three days, during which she walked, squatted, rocked by the fire, crouched, knelt, slept when contractions stopped, ate, sang, danced, lay in a hot tub 'in silent bliss' and sometimes at night walked around outside and counted the stars. She valued having friends and her older child with her to share the experience. This is how she describes what happened in the second stage:

> Together we proceeded to perform the incredible feat of pushing out a 10-pound baby. One friend held the camera, the midwives held my legs and my perineum, another friend held the watch, another the oxygen mask and Peyton held her doll and yelled, 'Come quick! The baby's head is coming! The baby's head is coming!' Now that's support!

The place of birth

One of the biggest decisions is *where* you are going to have your baby. This does not have to be the conventional hospital setting. In most places there are other options and you may want to explore alternatives to hospital.

Everything else that happens, and the relationship you have with those caring for you, is affected by your choice of birth place.

Birth at home

You may be thinking of having your baby at home. This means that you will be cared for by a midwife, though in many countries a general practitioner may attend you too. The pros and cons of home birth vary in different areas according to back-up services available, and, of course, the skills and personalities of the individual midwife and doctor. But, in general terms, planned home birth, as distinct from accidental out-of-hospital birth, is safe for a healthy woman whose pregnancy has been straightforward. British studies show a perinatal mortality (stillborn babies and those who die shortly after birth) of between 4 and 5 per 1,000. The babies who die are usually those who suffer from congenital handicaps. In Britain and North America this perinatal mortality rate is half or less than half that of babies born in hospital. It is comparable to the perinatal mortality rate in Scandinavian countries and the Netherlands, where birth is safer than anywhere else in the world.[7]

Planned home births produce the smallest proportion of low-birth-weight babies. In an English study, 2.5 per cent of home-birth babies weighed less than 2,500 grams, compared with 18 per cent booked for delivery in hospital.[8] Babies born at home usually start out on life healthy and vigorous.

Many obstetricians are implacably opposed to home birth, however. It is true, as they usually point out, that many more mothers and babies survive childbirth today than in 'the bad old days' when nearly every woman had her babies at home. But when two statistical trends occur at the same time, this does not prove that one was the cause of the other. A perinatal epidemiologist has pointed out that many more people have TV sets than 50 years ago, when perinatal mortality rates were higher. But no one suggests that the rise in TV ownership has caused the reduction in the perinatal mortality rate.[9] Many socio-economic changes have occurred over the last 50 years which have contributed to improvements in women's health and safer childbirth. These include smaller families, readily available contraception, abortion when a severely handicapped fetus is diagnosed, better nutrition, more awareness of the effects of pollution – and its reduction in many areas – and increased public education about health. In Britain the perinatal mortality rate started to decline during the Second World War. This was well before most women had their babies in hospital and before the introduction of modern technology such as electronic fetal monitoring. It was a time when women were cared for by midwives rather than doctors, many of whom were away in the armed forces, and when a system of food rationing, and the distribution of welfare orange juice, vitamins and milk, meant that the vast mass of people, and pregnant women in particular, had better and more wholesome nutrition than ever before. It is even possible that more babies would survive birth if hospitals had never taken over childbirth.[10]

Since 1973, as a consequence of a policy of hospitalization for all (about which women were never consulted), the proportion of out-of-hospital births which are accidental has become larger. As a result the mortality rate for home births appears to have risen compared with mortality rates in hospital. Deliveries in taxis, for example; the concealed births of babies to frightened teenagers, some of whom did not even know they were pregnant; births following illegal late abortions; those resulting from massive and sudden haemorrhage; and premature delivery of babies born long before a woman expected to go into labour – all these were classified as 'home' births. These *unplanned* (it might be better to call them 'uncared-for') births skew the statistics and result in uninformed general-izations about the risk of home birth.[11]

In Holland about a third of all babies are born at home – a higher proportion than in any other country in the Western world. The perinatal mortality for home births there was 3 per 1,000 in 1979. One study revealed that women who had home births experienced 'significantly fewer complications during pregnancy, delivery or puerperium than among those who had their babies in hospital'. Morbidity was also lower amongst babies born at home. The conclusion reached was that 'it is a responsible decision for a normal healthy woman given the right kind of antenatal supervision to have her baby at home . . .'[12]

If you decide that you want to give birth at home it may be difficult to find a doctor who will agree to it. Doctors have most or all of their training in hospital. Many have never seen a truly natural birth, without any intervention, and the absence of an institutional support system arouses anxiety. They are also often concerned about the attitudes of colleagues and of those higher up in the medical hierarchy. Even British general practitioners who have done home births in the past are increas-ingly nervous about agreeing to them, because they feel they are out of practice.

In the USA physicians worry about malpractice insurance and pos-sible litigation if things go wrong. Medical insurance companies refuse to insure a family practitioner who does home births and some refuse to insure any doctor who works with a midwife. Even in Britain, where there is much less litigation, doctors may give their worry about this as a reason for refusing to do home births. So having a baby at home may mean (especially in North America) that you have to forget about doctors and find a midwife.

An overwhelming advantage of home birth is that you control the territory in which birth takes place, and those helping you are guests in your home. You can move around just as you want, eat and drink, take a bath or go out for a walk – do whatever you feel like doing. You can have just your partner and the midwife with you, or a group of friends and family to whom you feel especially close, without having to ask permission. Your other children can be there too and, because it is home, can go in and out of the room freely. As one woman explained:

> Last time, the hospital atmosphere was very unsupportive. There were a load of routines and different kinds of interference which were never explained and I didn't have any choice about it. I'd already laboured happily

six hours at home, but from the moment I stepped inside that hospital I became a patient. Labour turned into an ordeal. Next time I want to be able to do whatever I feel like – eat when I want, labour in the bath, have the room dark, and groan and moan and yell and not be told over and over again that I need an epidural.

For two other women the reasons they chose home births were slightly different. One said:

I chose home birth mainly because it was a way I could get a VBAC (vaginal birth after a previous Caesarean section). No doctor in the area where I live would consider it. I feel, too, that birth should be a normal part of family life, and siblings are not allowed in the delivery rooms at either of the hospitals here.

The other woman focused mainly on the baby's birth experience:

I am concerned to make it as good as I can for the baby. The decisive thing was that I don't want my baby taken away from me at all, not even for a paediatric check or anything. I don't want any kind of drug going through the cord into the baby either, or in my breast milk afterwards. I'd like the delivery to be gentle and the baby always to be handled lovingly. The only way I can get that in this city is at home.

Disadvantages of home birth are that it may be difficult to find a doctor or midwife to attend you and even if you do you may be uncertain of his or her skills. (In the USA and Canada, a midwife may have no medical back-up, a disadvantage if problems develop.) You cannot have an epidural at home, and since that is the most effective form of pain relief, it is vital that you have other non-pharmacological ways of handling pain. Similarly, at home you cannot get the baby born by Caesarean section. If your labour is prolonged, or the baby's heart rate shows it is under special stress, or you bleed heavily afterwards, you have to be moved to hospital. Rarely – but it does happen sometimes – a baby has to be transported to special care.

You can find out more about home birth by reading my book *Birth at Home* (OUP, 1979) and some of the others in the reading list on pp. 308–9, and by contacting the home birth organizations listed on p. 313.

> Think through the pros and cons of home birth from your own point
> of view. Make a note of questions you would like to ask to get further
> information. If you decide that you want to give birth at home, work
> out a strategy for achieving this.

Birth centres, GP units and birthing rooms

A birth centre in North America is rather like a small cottage
hospital, but one that does births only. As a general rule it encourages
natural birth without medical intervention, has a warm, homely atmosphere and offers family-centred care, based on the principle that birth is
not a medical procedure but a natural physiological process in which a
woman benefits from loving human support. A birthing room is a labour–
delivery room within a hospital in which the same principles of care apply.
Birth centres and birthing rooms are springing up all over North America
and represent a radical innovation.

Birth centres are of two main types, either part of a larger hospital or
separate. Those outside hospitals may be within the medical system. Or
they may be right outside that system, having grown out of community-
based self-help and the initiatives of independent midwives. Because birth
centres cater for natural births only, there may be very careful screening
before a woman is allowed to book into one. Any whisper of difficulties
and she is transferred to a hospital. Some birth centres won't take women
over 35, or even those having a first baby, for example. Many are not
happy about accepting a woman who smokes in pregnancy.

In Britain small maternity hospitals corresponding to birth centres
and called 'general practitioner units' have been in existence for a long
time. Far from being regarded as the latest thing in health care, GP units
have often been closed on economic grounds and resources concentrated
in consultant units in large hospitals. Groups of women around the
country are fighting to save such GP units as still exist.

In GP units community midwives care for women and work closely
with GPs. This contrasts with the way midwives have to work in consultant units, where they are part of a team headed by the obstetrician.

In birth centres, GP units and birthing rooms, a woman usually
labours and delivers in the same room. You can bring in your own
cassette tape-recorder, pictures and other familiar objects you want to

have around you. Many of the rooms are quite cosy, with curtains, patterned wallpaper, hanging plants, a rocking chair, a carpet on the floor and soft lighting.

For women who have no serious problems in pregnancy, and who therefore do not need a high level of sophisticated care, births in this type of maternity unit – even when they are distant from hospital – are as safe as in units with a great deal of technology and obstetric intervention. Since GP units are an integral part of the National Health Service in Britain, much of the research has been done there.[13] It has been discovered that a midwife and family doctor actually provide better care for 'low-risk' women than that offered by specialized obstetricians. In a system with midwife care and home visits, women have fewer inductions, are less likely to be admitted in 'false labour', have reduced need of drugs for pain relief (and are more likely to have none at all), have fewer forceps deliveries and are less likely to have a perineal wound. Their babies tend to start to breathe earlier than those born in high-tech units and breastfeeding tends to be more successful.[14]

The idea behind hospital-based birth centres and birthing rooms is that there should be quick and easy access to obstetric skills and equipment when necessary. The problem is that in birth centres in large hospitals the transfer rate tends to be very high, mostly on the principle of 'just in case'. Even when a woman has got through the fine mesh of the screening process to be admitted to the birth centre in the first place, there is a strong probability that she will be 'wheeled down the corridor'. In some hospitals the care-givers she has chosen can stay with her. In others, there is a switch-over of staff at this point. From a woman's point of view it is obviously much better if she has the same people with her throughout. On the other hand, when it is simple for staff to transfer a woman to high-tech care – or even introduce it into the birthing room itself – while they still remain in charge, this is likely to happen the moment the midwife or doctor feels anxious that the labour is going on a long time, there is a lull in the activity of the uterus or the baby is not lying in a perfect position.

So one of the things you will probably want to find out if you are interested in a birth centre or birthing room within a hospital is the policy that controls care given there. Is there a time-limit on the first stage of labour, so that if dilatation progresses slowly, or you come to a sticking point when nothing seems to be happening, you are automatically moved? And will this in turn mean that you encounter a sudden staff change and have to cope with strangers at a point when everything seems to be going wrong? Or is there a flexible policy which takes into consideration a variety of patterns of labour which do not all conform to the textbook norm? If staff are equipped for high-tech intervention, such as the kind of electronic fetal monitoring which entails putting a clip on the baby's scalp, intravenous drips which stimulate the uterus, and epidural anaesthesia, in what percentage of women using the centre or room are these techniques employed? The answer to that question, if it is accurate, will give you a clear idea of the amount of intervention which a woman hoping for natural birth can anticipate. If a woman is transferred to another part of the hospital when there appear to be deviations from the normal, can her midwife continue to attend her, even if responsibility is taken over by the high-tech team?

Where a hospital has only a few birthing rooms (sometimes only one) you may find that when you happen to be in labour they are already occupied and you are forced to use the ordinary labour and delivery rooms. This does not matter a bit if the only difference between the birthing rooms and the rest of the hospital is one of interior decoration. It matters a lot if policy and the attitudes of care-givers are different.

In some hospitals the attitudes and atmosphere of the birthing rooms or birth centre, or in Britain of the integrated GP unit, have spilled over to the rest of the hospital, changed practice and reduced intervention, resulting, for example, in encouragement and emotional support being given in place of pain-killing drugs, and in lower rates of episiotomy and forceps delivery. In fact, in some British hospitals midwives are keen *not* to have special birthing rooms because they believe changes need to take place right through the hospital, and should not be limited to those women who want natural birth and are classified as 'low-risk'.

You cannot tell for sure whether a hospital has the atmosphere you are seeking simply from the presence of birthing rooms. Decor and furnishings are an insufficient guide to attitudes. There are hospitals where women are offered flowery curtains, patchwork quilts, a special birthing bed or chair and soft music, but where all this is merely a facade to interventionist obstetric practice. In countries such as the USA and Australia, where medical care is provided commercially – another commodity competing in the open market – hospitals provide these pleasant rooms to persuade women not to have their babies in rival hospitals or at home. Such competition may be a force for change but it can also result in 'window-dressing', with no real change in attitudes.

Make a note of the questions you want to ask administrators about facilities available in your area. It is a good idea to jot down the actual phrases you want to use and, in case replies are vague, any follow-up questions aimed at getting more specific answers.

You will probably want to talk to women who have had babies in these places, too. Decide what you want to focus on in your discussions with them and make a note of these subjects.

Here are the results of some women's investigations into birthing rooms and birth centres which they are considering:

DIANA (in Canada)

The hospital has a natural birth room. You can have up to four people with you, including your other children. If you want your children there, they must have an adult to look after them, and this must be someone other than your support person. They don't usually do shaves and enemas. You can walk around during labour and use the shower. Pethidine is given if drugs for pain relief are needed, but no epidural is available. Intravenous drips, oxytocin, electronic fetal monitoring and forceps are not used. After the birth, my partner could stay for up to 24 hours. However, very few births take place in the birth room – last year only 3 per cent of all vaginal births.

FRANKIE (in California)

This is a community-based birth centre in which lay midwives work. Most of those having their babies there are very poor Mexican women. The birth centre offers a package of prenatal care, nutritional counselling, care during birth and contraceptive advice. There isn't any emergency equipment to deal with complications. It is an ordinary house, with small birthing rooms, and there are usually not more than one or two women in labour at the same time. They are encouraged to move around in labour and can give birth in any position they like. The baby's father, other children, and relatives and friends can be there for the birth.

KATY (in London)

The hospital has a new birthing room which is very beautifully equipped and looks luxurious. There is TV, stereo, a bidet, indirect lighting, a rocking cradle. Electronic fetal monitoring is used for about 20 minutes after you are admitted and then for 15 minutes every hour. Many women have intravenous drips set up because they don't let you eat during labour. The baby's father or one other person can be with you. You can walk around when the fetal monitor is not being used. Analgesia is often given, but epidurals are not done in this room. The couple can have up to two hours with their baby after the birth.

Birth chairs and beds

Another option that may be available is a special birth chair or birthing bed. This is often rather like a dentist's chair and allows you to be in an upright position for delivery, if it is tilted at the right angle or has a squatting bar in place at the time. There is, however, no question of completely free movement, and you are more or less fixed and immobilized in it. Still, it is a great advance on the narrow, cold slab of the delivery table with its lithotomy stirrups (in which a woman's legs are fixed wide apart) and, in North America, handcuffs and shoulder restrainers. In fact, most of these birth chairs and beds have lithotomy stirrups too, but you don't usually see them when taken on a conducted tour. The firms manufacturing them make a particular point that they can be quickly adapted to enable staff to do obstetric operations and perform a wide range of manoeuvres. At least one birthing chair also has shoulder restrainers, so that the woman is firmly fixed in position and cannot move away from the obstetrician's hands if a painful intervention is performed.

Many women who have used birth chairs, especially if they had to lie on a delivery table for a previous birth, say that it made it much easier to push the baby out. They were more comfortable and it was good to be face-to-face with those caring for them, rather than lying on their backs staring up at powerful lights.

Most birth chairs are designed for the mother to sit, well supported, legs apart and knees bent. The mechanism to change the angle and the position of the footrests may be under her own control, but is often constructed to be controlled by attendants. If a chair is available and you think that you will want to adjust it yourself, look to see if you will be able to reach the control buttons.

Some chairs are very narrow so that it is difficult to spread yourself and to tilt your pelvis, for example, to adopt a position in which one knee is

4a   A birth chair.

4b   A birth chair
with squatting bar.
This allows more mobility.

bent while the other leg is extended. It can also be hard to straighten your legs, which you may want to do in between pushes. If you get a chance, it is a good idea not only to look at what is available, but actually to get on it and find out how it feels as you act through part of the second stage of labour. Imagine that you have bad backache, or that you are very uncomfortable with the baby's head like a huge melon pressing against your anus, and think how you may want to move then. Or imagine you have cramp in your leg and see if it is easy to extend your leg and foot, press the heel down on the foot support and rub your calf with one hand. Another point to check is whether you can bend forward easily, rounding your lower back, to see the top of your baby's head and stroke it if you wish. Some chairs are designed so that it is difficult to move your back freely. The moulded plastic fixes you in one position. There is one well-known chair in which it is impossible to rock your pelvis unless you press your feet into the footrests and stand up, gripping the sides of the chair.

Two obstetricians reporting on birth chairs in the *American Journal of Obstetrics*,[15] say that women who are in them for a long time tend to have oedema of the vulva, a condition they rarely met before they had a birth chair. They claim that this necessitates a large episiotomy, which heals poorly. So they insist on a woman being horizontal while she pushes – thus negating the whole idea of the birth chair, that a woman should be upright, in a physiologically correct and comfortable position. There have also been reports of heavy bleeding. Both oedema and bleeding result from immobility of the pelvis when the woman's position is fixed with her buttocks and thighs pressed against a hard, unyielding surface. So it is important to be free to move.

Another thing you may want to investigate is the material with which the chair is covered. Does it feel pleasant to the skin? Many women get very hot in the second stage of labour. Will the material feel comfortable if you are already hot? Is it slippery? Find out whether your body will be in direct contact with it, or whether a sheet, some towelling or a pillow is used as well.

A birth chair or bed is usually placed under a bright light for delivery. It is distressing for a woman to have a light shining in her eyes right through the second stage. Will it be possible to give birth in soft light, or at least to have a bright light only on your perineum? Ask to see how the lighting can be modified.

If you have the chance of using a birth chair or bed, make a checklist in your notebook. These are some of the items you may want to cover:

Can I get into squatting position if I wish?
Upright position?
Freedom for pelvic movement.
Comfortable support for back.
Is there something of the right height and angle to hold on to while in different positions?
Easily accessible controls which can be self-operated.
Range of variation of angles for back and leg support.
Texture of material used for covering.
Position of lighting and whether it can be modified.

There may be other equipment available which you would like better than a chair or bed. If it is not provided by the hospital, you may be able to take it in yourself.

A large beanbag or floor cushion can be comfortable to sit up against or to lean forward on to in a kneeling position if you have backache. You can use it either on a bed or on the floor.

A low stool gives support for a squatting position. It can be of the kind used by a small child to reach the lavatory, or the sort of stool provided in hospital to climb on to a high bed or delivery table. Or it may be a special birth stool, shaped like a horseshoe or boomerang, similar to those used by midwives throughout the Middle Ages. Some of these have a back. They limit mobility of the pelvis, and some are so high that you cannot squat. Choose one which does not slip on a tiled floor; rubber knobs over the feet can make it more stable. A stool should not be used on a delivery table. You don't feel safe and you could fall.

If you choose a stool, your support person can sit behind you on a higher chair, legs apart, cradling you against his or her body. Or you can have a big cushion or a wall behind you so that you can lean back between contractions.

A towel or sheet knotted to any strong bar, so that you can pull on it from a squatting position, may feel right. Fifty or 60 years ago women often gave birth pulling on a strip of material tied to a door or a bed-post. Or you can sit on a bucket with a towel folded on the rim under your buttocks. Many women find it easiest to push when they are sitting on the lavatory, and this position is similar.

5a Using a birth stool
with the birth
companion cradling
the woman in
his arms and
providing support
with his thighs.

5b Another position
using a birth stool,
with the birth
companion giving
firm back pressure.
Many women like
to move between
these two positions.

In the second stage of labour a woman often feels she needs to get her feet planted firmly on the floor. She feels most secure this way and physiological coordination comes most naturally. She may want to grip a piece of furniture which is handy or hold on to the person who is helping her. In many British hospitals women can now give birth on a sterile sheet on the floor. Sometimes this is placed over a mattress. In this way the

6a   A supported squatting position
for the second stage of labour.
It is important not to press hard underneath the woman's arms
because this can cause temporary nerve damage.

woman is not fixed in one position. She can move freely, changing position whenever she wants. The midwife kneels or sits beside her and delivers the baby from the front, back or side, as the mother wishes. In at least one hospital all midwives wear tracksuits so that they can do this easily.

Freedom of movement is important to give the best chance of a spontaneous vaginal delivery, especially if labour is difficult and the second

6b   A variation on the
supported squatting position
in which the birth companion grasps the woman's wrists.

stage long drawn out, with the baby in an awkward position, or with a tight fit between the baby's head and the maternal pelvis.

Expensive equipment is not necessary for comfort in childbirth. Nowadays an elaborate birth chair is sometimes provided as if it could guarantee the right conditions for natural birth. It doesn't. It may even be available mainly to deflect any further questions women may have about natural birth. It is as if the hospital is saying: 'Look at the amount of money we have spent to provide the latest model in birth chairs. This is evidence that we encourage women to give birth naturally. What else can you want?' The answer to that is – freedom of movement. Most hospitals have a very long way to go before that is achieved.

When you think about making your plans for birth, a vital element is deciding on an environment that would be right for you. This does not simply involve a choice between home and hospital; there are many options to consider in organizing a setting in which you will be able to feel relaxed and confident.

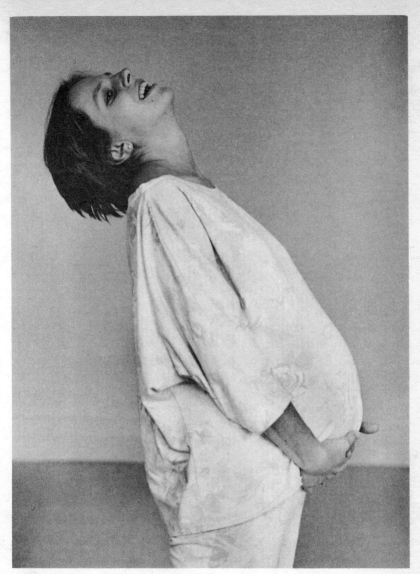

Ripe with Child

12

GETTING IN TOUCH
WITH YOUR BABY

You may veer between imagining your baby in every detail and thinking that a mass of moving limbs can't possibly be a baby at all: it must be an octopus or a basket of kittens. On quiet days it may feel like an awkward bump or inanimate doll or you forget all about it. Then there is a sudden burst of activity and you are fully aware that there is a living being waiting to burst into the world.

Pregnancy is a time not only for getting ready for childbirth, but also for preparing to be a mother, with all the powerful emotions this involves. Some women prefer to leave these emotions to take care of themselves:

> I'm too busy for introspection. I hope I'll be an adequate mother. But with the heavy load of teaching I'm doing this year there is no time now.

Other women enjoy this emotional journey to motherhood:

> I don't think I could ever be a 'Madonna mother', calm and tender all the time. But I'm sure I can be a stimulating mother and the baby will be fascinating to watch grow and develop. Sometimes I panic that I have no maternal instinct. Then the baby moves, I put my hand on the bump and it feels magical and I realize I shan't have to struggle to produce the right emotions. They're all there!

A woman needs time to get in touch with her baby and with her changing self, to dream and let fantasies play around the idea of the coming baby. This is not self-indulgence. It is not time wasted. It is an important part of preparing for the new relationship with another human being.

The ancient Chinese dated an individual life from nine months before birth. Nowadays a new science of perinatal psychology is developing which explores the influences on a baby which can operate prenatally, during birth and immediately following delivery.

To some women this may seem another burden placed on them, a duty to make contact with the fetus, concentrate on it and consider its needs – at the expense of their own. This imposes additional stress on pregnancies which are often stressful anyway. A woman has her own needs, her own priorities and rights, and they are not all subsumed by the fact that she is going to have a baby. That is one compelling reason why the exercise of choice about what she does in pregnancy is vital.

On the other hand, increased awareness of the baby inside, making contact with it, is for some women an enhancement of pregnancy:

> It's one of the things I enjoy about being pregnant – feeling the baby move and talking to it. It's a different rhythm of living. Usually it's all rush and go. I've calmed down. I'm turned inward.

Even for a woman who can't afford time to slow down – who is, for example, especially busy in her job, perhaps trying to clear the decks in order to take maternity leave – a break in her hectic life when she focuses on the baby can be refreshing and restful. For some women it is a luxurious interlude in the last three months of pregnancy.

Life before birth

The fetus cannot respond to stimuli until it has developed a nervous system which makes this possible. Consciousness demands something else again: the nerve pathways which allow the cerebral cortex, the part of the brain which is necessary for thought, to function are not connected till after the beginning of the 28th week of pregnancy (dating it from the first day of the mother's last period).[1]

Reflex activities, however, start long before that. They occur spontaneously and can also be stimulated by touching the fetus. As early as 13 weeks the fetus moves its tongue and can swallow. In another week lip movements begin and it is capable of facial expressions.

From about 10 weeks the amniotic fluid in which the fetus is lying flows into its open mouth and by at least 15 weeks it can distinguish different tastes. Amniotic fluid contains traces of sugar, various acids, protein, mineral salts, fat and so on.[2] Taste preferences seem to be already established in the uterus, since studies done with newborn babies reveal that they suck more quickly when fed sweet fluids and sucking is slower and they grimace when fed fluids containing quinine or citric acid.[3] Babies also prefer sweet to plain water. Not only do they suck more strongly, but their heart rates speed up.[4] They like plain water better than salt water and are very quick to notice salt, even in low concentrations.[5]

What the baby can hear

Already by 10 weeks the vestibular (balancing) system is functioning. The fetus can orient itself in space.

Back in the mid-seventies medical researchers examining the results of studies of fetal response to sound concluded: 'It is clear that long before birth, the fetus can hear and respond to sound and that the uterus is not a soundproof chamber.'[6] Since that time the ultrasound scan and fetal heart monitor, whatever disadvantages and hazards they may have when used routinely in pregnancy and birth, have produced increased understanding of life inside the uterus, of what the fetus can hear, and even its preferences.

The ear is the only part of the body to reach adult size while the baby is still inside the uterus. At 12 weeks the nerve endings necessary for hearing develop. By 20 weeks the complex, fluid-filled labyrinth of the inner ear is formed and the baby responds to various kinds of sound, though until about 32 weeks this sound is not transmitted in the same way that it is after delivery. The fetus can respond to resonance, however, long before it can hear clearly. This may be why fetal movements and increased heart rates are recorded at four to five months when music is played. Babies at this stage can distinguish between different kinds of music, becoming more active when Beethoven and Brahms are played and calming down in response to Vivaldi and Mozart.[7]

Even when the baby does not actually move to music, its heart rate changes. Loud sound produces a quicker heart rate. Babies probably cannot hear anything below 40 decibels.[8] David Chamberlain, a psychologist who has done a great deal of work on consciousness at birth and on birth memories, points out: 'This puts many of the sounds in the baby's natural environment clearly within audible range.'[9]

The baby inside its mother's body can also pick up the frequencies of human speech. In fact, it appears to store speech patterns learnt from its mother. Babies move their bodies and eyes in a pattern which is synchronized with the speech of whoever is talking to them. They do not do this if presented with a gabble of speech sounds, only with language.[10] They respond in this way whether the language is English or Chinese.[11] So it seems that in the last months of pregnancy, once hearing is developed, the baby, though lying in water in which sound is picked up differently from sound carried in air, is already 'tracking' human speech and being acculturated to the tones and rhythms of the language spoken by its mother.

A newborn baby can recognize its mother's voice. Given a choice between her voice and another female voice the baby will opt for the mother's. In one experiment babies less than four days' old were given a rubber teat to suck which did not provide milk.[12] By changing their sucking rate the babies could get the recorded voice of their own mother reading a Dr Seuss story or the same story read by another woman. In less than 20 minutes the babies learnt how to get their mothers. If there are other children in the family the fetus almost certainly hears and responds to their voices too. Young children's voices are even higher pitched than the mothers', and because 2- and 3-year-olds are usually in close proximity to the mother, sitting on her lap, being cuddled, climbing over her – and can also be very noisy – it would be surprising if the fetus did not become familiar with the sound of its siblings' voices. In my own experience the newborn can often be comforted by the sound of its siblings' voices and becomes quietly attentive.

The baby also practises muscle movements which, once it is born, produce a cry – and for each baby that cry is as unique as a fingerprint. To anybody who has not had a baby, different babies' cries may sound very similar, but any mother knows she can pick out her own baby amid a dozen or so others. This cry has been rehearsed already in the uterus and was in turn derived from her speech pattern.[13]

Within a few minutes of birth a baby turns its head in the direction of a sound, particularly that of the human voice,[14] and prefers the high-pitched sound of a woman's speech to the lower pitch of a man's. Many people spontaneously speak at a higher pitch when talking to new babies. In a tape recording of one of my own children's births, my husband first speaks to me in his normal voice and then turns to his newborn daughter and says, in a noticeably higher-pitched voice, 'Hello! What are we going to call you, little one?'

The fetus can hear the churning of the mother's digestive system and the pulsing of blood through her arteries and veins. There is also the steady drumming of her heart-beat. The sound of the human heart seems to be particularly comforting to newborn babies. In a well-known study, the sound of a heart beating at 72 beats per minute was played to babies in a hospital nursery.[15] There was a control group of babies who did not hear the sound. The babies' crying in the two nurseries was recorded and their milk intake and weight gain were measured over a period of four days. The babies in the control group cried nearly twice as much as those in the heart-beat group. Twice as many babies in the heart-beat group put on weight, though each set of babies was taking approximately the same quantity of milk. Those who were soothed by the sound of the heart-beat seemed to be able to make better use of the food.

When the heart-beat was speeded up to 128 beats per minute none of the babies liked it and they all started crying. So it is not just any noise that works, but specifically a sound to which the baby has become accustomed in the uterus and which represents closeness to the mother and security with her.

Sleeping and waking

Already by the fifth month of pregnancy the baby has its own pattern of sleep and waking. In the last three months of pregnancy there are some times when the baby seems to exercise strenuously and others when it is alert and there is a potential for movement in response to sound, the mother's change of position, or hand pressure on the abdominal wall. It is particularly in this state of waking that she can get in contact with her baby. It corresponds to the 'quiet, alert' state which psychologists have described in the new born baby, a time when the baby catches the parents' attention and they can have a 'conversation'.

Sleeping periods are of two distinct kinds, too. During REM sleep rapid eye movements occur. This is dreaming sleep. Non-REM sleep is deep sleep in which the heart rate is slower and the eyes do not move. At 30 weeks a baby spends its entire sleeping time in REM sleep. By 33 to 35 weeks this has been reduced to 67 per cent of the time, by 36 to 38 weeks it is 38 per cent and at 40 weeks, when the baby is ready to be born, half its time is spent in REM sleep.[16] The fetus often moves during REM sleep and is apparently moving in response to a dream. The authors of this research believe that dreaming sleep is important for the final development of the central nervous system and, in later life, for its maintenance.

The definite waking and sleeping cycle of the last few months of pregnancy is often similar to the pattern of waking and sleeping which exists following birth. The undrugged baby usually has a period of alertness after delivery. It lasts for an hour or two, but then the baby sleeps for much of the time for the next three to four days. As the mother's breast-milk comes in there are more frequent waking periods and there tend to be one or two prolonged waking times during the 24 hours. A baby who kicked regularly every evening while inside the uterus is likely to have an evening waking time afterwards. One common waking period is between 8.00 p.m. and 11.00 p.m. For many babies it is longer than that. Just as the mother wants to have some peace and quiet at the end of the day, the baby wakes up.

> When you are in the last 10 weeks of your pregnancy make a note of the times when your baby is most active over a period of a week. See if any pattern emerges.

Harriet's baby, Dan, is now five months old. Looking back to what she learnt about him before he was born, she says:

> In the morning he was quiet, though I may have thought that because I was so busy and didn't notice when he moved. Early afternoon was a kicking time. But he kicked more after six in the evening. Sometimes he kicked so much that I felt quite bruised under my ribs. And now he always sleeps solidly in the morning, which lets me get on with things. Then he likes a playtime after lunch, has a nap after that, and then his main waking time is from about six in the evening till about 10.30. It's very difficult to get him to settle before that. I start the evening meal before he wakes up and David finishes it. Then I eat while he holds Dan. Then I hold him while he eats. We switch the record player on and sometimes we put him in the baby sling and we dance! Our evenings are very energetic.

Movement clues

A healthy fetus moves a lot right up to the time of birth, though mothers' awareness of movements varies a good deal. One woman may consistently record few movements and another always record a great many. Movements change at different phases of pregnancy too. When they are first felt at 18 to 20 weeks they feel like small nudges, like bubbles popping, or as if a bird has fluttered its wings inside you. Later they turn into obvious bumps and knocks. From 19 weeks the baby begins to make breathing movements as if in rehearsal for breathing after birth. These movements get stronger and occur more often, until by 27 weeks they form a regular rhythm of activity.

Until 24 to 26 weeks the baby has enough room to turn complete somersaults. Within the next four to six weeks it usually turns head down (termed 'vertex' or 'cephalic' presentation) into the position for birth. The head is the largest and heaviest part and usually fits neatly in the cavity of the bony pelvis like an egg in an egg-cup. Because it is a tight fit it stays there, and is then said to be 'engaged'.

From that stage on the baby can switch from side to side, rotate its head and swing its whole body round, but can no longer change position so that it is bottom down.

There are several distinct kinds of movement which you may be able to distinguish in the last months of pregnancy. One is the body roll. The baby turns from one side of the abdomen to the other, and then perhaps back again. At the height of the action there is a momentary pause as your abdomen is pushed out by the hard curve of the baby's back. It sticks out like the shell of a giant turtle.

Another movement comes from the feet, which you may feel kicking up under your ribs on the left or right side. The baby's body is on the opposite side to where you can feel the kicking. If you are aware of these foot movements you can be sure that the baby is head down and anterior, that is with the back of its head towards your front. The firm, melon-shaped curve at the front is the baby's back. This is an excellent position for the baby to be in when labour starts.

The baby is born with a reflex to bend its knee up when pressure is applied to the sole of the foot. In late pregnancy the walls of the upper part of the uterus become thicker as part of a process in which the lower segment gets thinner and muscle fibres are drawn up into the top of the uterus. The baby's feet are pressing against this strong wall. When the uterus contracts, as it does regularly, pressure is exerted on the feet. This encourages the baby to make the stepping movements which you feel as kicks. They help the baby to curl up in a ball, with limbs flexed, back rounded and its head forward on its chest. This position has a mechanical advantage in labour because when the uterus tightens it can press the ball of the baby's head down through the open cervix and the curve of the birth canal.

You may also feel the baby bouncing its head. This only happens when it has engaged. The baby is born with a reflex to lift its chin when pressure is exerted against the top of its head. Your pelvic floor muscles lie across the outlet of the bony pelvis beneath the baby's head. Every now and again the baby bounces its head against them, using them rather like a trampoline. For you the sensation is one of tingling in your vagina as if you were being tickled or having a very mild electric shock. With this head movement the baby helps itself wriggle deeper into a good position for birth, head tucked firmly against the cervix, the part of the uterus which is going to open in labour.

You may also sometimes experience quick staccato movements. They may be hiccups. Or they may be the rapid movements of the baby's head from side to side in order to find again a thumb or finger which it was sucking but has lost for a moment. After birth this rooting reflex helps the baby find the nipple.

By the end of pregnancy the baby rarely goes ten minutes without moving in some way, simply practising breathing movements – which you cannot feel – or bending or stretching an arm or leg, waving, kicking, turning or rolling from one side to the other – and the bigger the movement the more likely you are to feel it.[17]

In late pregnancy many women discover that it is possible to affect the baby's behaviour, to send a message so that it moves or quietens down, for example. It may get into a position which is uncomfortable for you, with a foot sticking in your ribs. Try shifting your position or pressing a hand firmly over the baby's back to get it to roll into a different position. A very active baby who is twisting and dipping, turning and bumping, can often be calmed by a hand cupped over its buttocks, by slow, deep breathing or with soft music. A baby often seems especially active just as the mother is trying to go to sleep and she learns that changing her position, cradling its back between her hands and telling it to quieten down can soothe it.

A woman may also discover that the baby reacts to certain kinds of sound, apparently getting excited by some or becoming still and even going to sleep in response to others.

She may be aware, too, that her own emotional state affects the baby. If she is feeling lazy and soporific as she lies in the sun on a beautiful summer day, movements often slow down and become spaced further apart. If she grabs a few minutes to rest during a very busy day, however, the baby is likely to be churning around as if it were aware of all the rush and bustle and the host of things on her mind.

When women start to relax and breathe slowly in childbirth classes, babies usually move energetically at first. This seems to be a response to the mother starting to let go the tensions she felt about getting to the class, leaving work on time, making a meal, organizing the family, making sure her partner is ready, manoeuvring through traffic to get across town, and so on. When she has settled down into rhythmic, full breathing and feels relaxed, the baby slows down too.

Fetal Behaviour [18]

8 weeks The embryo starts to make tiny movements and may get hiccups, but the mother cannot feel these yet.

9 weeks Starts to kick.

10 weeks Moves more than 12 per cent of the time, also begins to make breathing movements, and now or in a couple of weeks starts to drink amniotic fluid.

11 weeks Movements become more vigorous. Occasionally jumps as if startled.

12 weeks In response to stimulus, closes its mouth and swallows.

13 weeks Bouts of hiccups most frequent at this stage of pregnancy. When the fetus hiccups it does so 26 to 28 times a minute.

16 weeks Has developed a sense of taste. In experiments the fetus doubles its swallowing rate if amniotic fluid is artificially sweetened. If a bright light is shone on the mother's abdomen the heart rate speeds up and it turns its head away.

18 weeks Movements are first felt by the mother now or within the next three weeks.

20 weeks If the fetus touches something, it grasps it and moves its arm up and down.

22 weeks From now on the heart rate speeds up when the fetus moves and it also begins to make definite sucking movements.

25 weeks May react to loud, sudden noises, become quiet when the mother speaks softly, and fall asleep when she walks around and it is rocked in the cradle of her pelvis.

27 weeks Makes strong breathing movements now.

28 weeks At about this time the brain has developed to a point where it can be assumed that there is consciousness.

29 weeks The baby responds to sound by moving more and its heart-beat gets faster.

30 weeks The baby's experience of its own heart-beat seems to be important from now on for establishing a response to rhythm after birth.

33 weeks From now on there are two states of sleep: rapid eye movement (REM) or active sleep, which in adults is dreaming sleep, and deep, non-REM sleep.

37 weeks By now the baby moves in some way at least every 10 minutes. Some of these movements cannot be felt by the mother because it is breathing activity, which occurs in spurts.

39 weeks During quiet sleep the baby often makes mouth movements at 10- to 20-second intervals. In active sleep the baby moves every 0.5 to 2.5 minutes and makes sucking and other mouth movements for 5 seconds to 3 minutes. At this stage of pregnancy the baby spends 95 per cent of the time asleep.

The baby's position

As you get near the end of pregnancy you can discover how your baby is lying by feeling the different parts of its body through your abdominal wall. The obstetric term for this is 'palpation'. The next time you see your obstetrician or midwife, you may want to ask them to show you how to do it.

Here is how you can start finding out how your baby is lying, in a way that is rather different from the medical method but which may work well for you.

Empty your bladder first, as this makes it easier to feel the different parts of the baby. Lie on your back propped up with pillows. Now have a

7a The baby is in an anterior position (in this case on the mother's left).

7b This baby, with knees bent, is a complete breech. When the baby's legs are drawn up like this it is easy for it to curl up into a ball and so travel through the pelvis.

look at the curve of your abdomen. Can you see any obvious bumps? Look especially around your navel. If it is popping out like a seam coming untucked you can be almost certain that, for the moment anyway, the baby is in an anterior position, with its back well to the front. If there is a slight dip around your navel or it is level, the baby is probably sideways-on at present. If there is a saucer-shaped dip it is likely to be posterior – lying facing your front. The space is the gap between its legs and arms. Give a long breath out and relax completely so that muscles are not tense and you can feel through them with your hands.

In the last few weeks your baby is most likely to be lying head down with its back more or less towards your front. So feel first whether the feet are under your ribs on the right or left side. Moving your hands slowly and deliberately, press in firmly. A foot feels rather like a small knob on an old-fashioned brass bedstead, or a knobbly door handle. You can often coax it to move by pressing it hard with your finger. If the baby is awake and it really is a foot it will be drawn away and then, perhaps, come back again. You will probably be able to feel an obvious foot shape and hold the baby's foot in your hands. If you cannot find the foot under your ribs but can feel kicking in the lower part of your abdomen it is very likely that your baby is head up in the uterus – breech.

7c A frank breech. When the legs are straight like this it is called an 'extended' or 'frank' breech. Descent may be slower than for a complete breech because the legs are splinting the baby's spine.

7d The baby is in a posterior position.

If you feel kicking all over your front and have a saucer-shaped dip by your navel, the baby is probably posterior at the moment. Its back is lying against your back. If the head has not yet dropped down into the pelvis the baby may change between anterior and posterior several times during the day. If the head has engaged, however, you may start labour with the baby in this position and contractions will press the head round into the more favourable anterior position. This often takes a long time. The mother gets backache because the hard back of the head is pressed against the small of her back. With patience the baby almost always turns. But if it has not turned it can be born as a posterior. This is a rather more difficult delivery as a wider part of the baby's head is coming through the birth canal. Obstetricians often turn the head with forceps, a ventouse (vacuum suction machine) or manually.

Both the head and the bottom are hard. But the head is round like a ball, whereas the bottom is flatter. To distinguish the head from the bottom you can try palpating what you think is its head. Place your fingers on each side of it and try to bounce the bump before your fingers. The head moves like a cork floating in water. The baby's bottom will not move. When the head is up under your ribs, it may feel rather like a small upturned saucepan sitting there uncomfortably. If the baby is head down and engaged you may not be able to feel the head at all because it is deep inside the pelvis.

7e The baby's head is engaged – i.e., the top of the head is at a level of the ischial (pronounced 'iskeeal') spines. It is at 'zero'.

7f The baby lying transverse.

Here are some clues to help you decide whether or not the baby's head has dipped into the pelvis. The head is likely to be engaged if:
   – when you stand you feel as if there is something heavy between your legs;
   – you are uncomfortable sitting down quickly on a hard chair;
   – you get an occasional 'buzzing' in your vagina as the baby bounces its head against your muscles;
   – you feel pressure against your bladder and have to empty it more often;
   – it is easier to breathe than it was a few weeks back as there is less pressure against your ribs;
   – the baby is no longer leaping about so much;
   – you can feel knobbly feet under your ribs;
   – you have located the baby's head in the lower part of your abdomen on previous occasions, but now you can't find anything you can identify as a head.

You can also use your hands to check whether the head is engaged. Place them just above the pubic bone at either side of the part of the baby's body you can feel there. Then walk your fingers in from the outer edge towards the middle. If there is a space at the bottom where your fingers can meet, between the rounded curve of the baby and the edge of your pubic bone, the head is not yet engaged. If there is no space at all, the head has engaged and the part of the baby's body you are tracking with your fingers is probably the shoulders.

Even if the baby is not engaged when you are lying down, it may become so when you stand up. You can feel it drop like a large orange and press against your bladder and vagina.

Second and subsequent babies often do not engage until just before you start labour, or even after it has already begun.

If your partner or a friend is feeling the baby's position, guide their hands and put your hands over theirs to give them confidence to press firmly enough and to show them the degree of pressure that feels comfortable for you – and don't forget to talk to the baby at the same time.

Sometimes the baby never fixes in one position. This often occurs when a woman has already had several previous pregnancies. In late pregnancy the baby then often lies across the uterus. If the baby is fixed in this position during labour it cannot come down the birth canal, but it usually turns and is head down by the very end of pregnancy, slipping deep into the pelvis when strong contractions start.

Dreaming

Especially at the very beginning and the end of pregnancy, many women find they dream a good deal. These dreams may be very vivid. Some women dream in colour, having only dreamed in black and white before. Many say that themes are repeated in different forms on several occasions or that they have various versions of the same dreams. Sometimes these are disturbing.

The baby is often represented as a baby animal – a kitten or puppy perhaps. Or it may be turned into a part of the body which has dropped off or been amputated. Sometimes it is a tooth which is extracted. This is not surprising, as during pregnancy it feels to the woman as if the baby were part of her own body – and birth brings with it the necessity of separation.

Water is an age-old symbol of birth. Sometimes dreams involving water express fear of birth and its danger. Sometimes, on the contrary, these water-dreams convey a sense of fulfilment.

Many women have dreams about being in hospital; sometimes these are nightmares. One woman who had had a previous distressing labour and then been separated from her baby, who was in the special-care nursery, had repeated dreams during her subsequent pregnancy of being tied down on the delivery table, with doctors and nurses wearing devils' masks and her baby inside a glass bottle.

Some dream of a machine which has started and cannot be stopped, a vivid symbol of the feeling a pregnant woman often has that she is taken over by doctors and the hospital system. Some have dreams of being trapped, behind a locked door, for example, perhaps because they feel powerless in the hands of professionals, or trapped by the pregnancy itself.

Women who already have children often have nightmares in which one of these is harmed because of their own negligence or inattention. 'I am going through the yard gate,' Carole said, 'and my 2-year-old is running in front of me and suddenly she darts right out into the road. There is a screech of tyres, a scream. The car stops. Her body lies there.' A woman often feels guilty that, with a new baby on the way, she is not giving enough love to the older child and her sense of guilt is expressed in dreams like this.

When a woman wakes in the night she may put it down to pressure on her bladder or the baby's movements, but these physical causes of waking can mask the stimulus of powerful and disturbing dreams. It seems simpler to explain the sudden waking in physical terms than to dredge up to the surface of consciousness exactly what happened in a dream. But sometimes tracking these dreams down and recollecting them can help to pin-point anxiety which has been unacknowledged. It is often useful to do this so that something can be done to defuse the anxiety.

It may be a matter of getting hold of more information, achieving better communication with care-givers, talking through something which is on your mind with someone close to you, or sharing with other women who have gone through a similar experience.

> You may want to jot down any pregnancy dreams which you feel throw some light on your hopes and fears or on things which are important to you about the birth and the baby.

Maternal emotions

When a pregnant woman is very frightened or angry, stress hormones flood into her bloodstream and through the placenta, so that her baby is transfused with them too. Most women notice how when they are alarmed, furiously angry or highly aroused in any way, the baby jumps around a great deal, and may go on being restless for an hour or more after they themselves have calmed down. Stress hormones seem to send an alarm signal to the baby to speed up its heart rate, and to provoke what feels to the mother like agitated behaviour.

But this is not the only way in which the baby may respond to our own violent emotions. If a woman is under great stress other metabolic changes occur too. Her breathing, her heart rate, blood pressure and state of muscle tension are all affected, and this in turn may affect her fetus.

Fear triggers a physical 'fight-or-flight' reaction. Blood flows to the large muscles so that we can resist attack or escape. In a pregnant woman the fight-or-flight reaction occurs at the expense of the blood supply to the uterus, so that the baby gets less oxygen. Most babies are pretty tough and can cope well with isolated incidents of this kind, but if the mother is under prolonged stress the baby's oxygen supply may be reduced for a long period.

Some psychotherapists claim that this can set up a pattern of emotion in the baby – panic, helplessness or depression, for example – which may stay with a person throughout life. They say that reliving incidents in our prenatal life and birth, with the pain and terror we felt then, can enable us to understand these feelings and cope with them better.[19] These psychologists believe that though the brain is important for memory retrieval, memory *storage* may take place through the whole cellular chemistry of the body. When people replay painful experiences which happened in the uterus or during birth, these memories, they say, can be picked up by the conscious mind and turned into words. Once they have become words, adults understand themselves better and use the experience to grow emotionally.

'A cynical part of myself,' a British psychoanalyst remarked, 'says that all this is just a useful symbol. But it is one everyone understands . . . we can all think back to being in a little capsule with one portal of entry, totally helpless and dependent, and then struggling out through a narrow exit.'

Knowing that the baby is a feeling creature, already learning inside the uterus, and that it can receive messages and even, in a rudimentary way, send messages to you, means that bonding between you both can start long before birth. When you can start on a relationship with your baby during pregnancy the whole process unfolds gradually. It is not, as it now sometimes seems to be in the delivery room, a sudden demand to bond and prove that you have the appropriate maternal feelings.

Being in touch with the baby inside has practical implications too. Not only do you become aware of your baby's rhythms of sleep and waking and the pattern of its movements, but you are probably the most reliable guide to your baby's well-being. Though many hospitals still rely on hormone tests of urine or blood to discover if the placenta is working properly in late pregnancy, when mothers themselves keep kick charts they are often more accurate in predicting problems than any chemical tests.[20]

Bearing in mind the stimuli to which the fetus is known to respond and the ways in which your emotional state may affect the baby, think now of other things you could do to get in touch with the baby inside you. Some of these may affect the baby through changes in your feelings, muscle tone and breathing, others through changes in posture or through sound. Here are some different activities you might choose:

Practise deep relaxation
Breathe slowly and completely
Sing
Play music
Walk energetically in the fresh air

Dance
Exercise with pelvic movements

In your notebook jot down anything you noticed concerning your baby's activity.

There are obvious hazards resulting from the new knowledge that babies in the uterus can feel and hear and that they have a developing awareness of their mothers and of the world into which they are going to be born. One of the psychologists at the Toronto Congress of Perinatal Psychology said that if the woman didn't want to be pregnant or hated her pregnancy, 'the child gets the message of fear and rejection and may feel that she isn't wanted, that she doesn't belong on the earth, through her entire life'. That kind of statement ignores the power of mammalian biology to provide a good deal of protection to the fetus through the exquisite mechanism of the placenta. In seeking to emphasize the closeness of the relationship between the mother and baby before birth, and criticizing the old idea of the uterus as a safe haven, it goes to the opposite extreme. This is likely to be just as inaccurate.

It is also a heavy burden to place on the mother. An involuntary, biological, instinctual power is ascribed to women in order to deny their rights as individuals and render them powerless. If we have this influence on our unborn babies through our blood and hormones it seems that the baby must be at the centre of all our thinking, and that we dare not express our true feelings. It can make pregnancy a kind of imprisonment. A woman is trapped with a being who has taken over her body and whom she is never allowed to ignore or forget. She has a duty to be happy right through the 24 hours, not for her own sake, but because if she lets herself be depressed or anxious, so she is told, she can damage her baby irreparably. If the child does not turn out well, it is all going to be *her fault*.

To be able to nurture and enjoy her baby spontaneously, in pregnancy as well as after the baby is born, a woman needs to be nurtured and cherished *herself*. If she feels secure and confident, supported by people who love her, and has a chance to get to know her baby in her own time, without feeling that she has to put on a performance, she spontaneously cares for her child in exactly the right way.

Closeness to the baby after birth

When the baby is born you may feel that at last you can belong to yourself again and be happy to put the baby down in a crib whenever you can and rediscover your own identity. But something else may happen. Even though you were weighed down with the baby in the last weeks of pregnancy and were looking forward to being able to reclaim your body, once the baby is born you may miss having it inside you and feel empty. If anyone insists on taking the baby away – even if only into another room – you experience an intense feeling of loss. It is only when the baby is close and in your arms that you feel really whole again. These powerful feelings serve an important biological function. They ensure that newborn babies are cared for, cuddled and fed and that the mother does this not just out of duty, but because she *longs* to do so.

As a woman gets to know her newborn baby she is caught up in a demanding and unremitting process. Babies need their nappies changed and their bottoms wiped. They have to be fed regularly and in the early weeks like to feed and suck ad lib. They may bring back milk and burp and fill their nappies again just after they have been changed. And when they need you – for food or comfort – they cry, and go on crying until that need is satisfied.

When you think about this in advance, or if you watch other parents servicing *their* babies, it may all seem rather offensive. You may hope that you can organize your life differently and regulate things so that your day does not revolve around the baby in such a demanding way. But the strange thing is that when you have your own baby, wanting to be separate and in control gives way to pleasure in closeness with the baby, finding what the baby wants and enjoying his or her dependence on you.

This change in your feelings affects decisions you'll make about whether, for example, you want to breast-feed or bottle-feed your baby. To have the baby in your own bed or in a separate room; to cuddle the baby close in a sling against your body or put her down in a pram for lengthy periods of time.

Most new mothers enjoy the feeling of the baby close to them, the smell of her skin, the rounded curve of the head, the firm weight of the little body in their arms. Even though a woman thought she had no 'maternal instincts' she usually, given half a chance, can't help falling in love with her baby.

One way of preparing yourself for this experience and getting in touch with your feelings is to take time to think, and, perhaps just as important, to *dream* and have fantasies, about holding your baby, cuddling and feeding it. Think how it would feel, for example, to have your child close to you in bed at night, a tiny hand gripping your finger, the weight of the head in the crook of your arm and the firm, rounded buttock in your hand, or to have the baby sucking at your breast, attached firmly as a limpet. Here is how some women imagine their feelings:

> A bit like the feeling I have with my cat. I like stroking her, she is so soft and furry and she purrs with pleasure. I have never thought of myself holding a baby but I know I enjoy cats and other baby animals.

> Sometimes it is almost as if Pete's like a baby. When we are relaxed I hold his head in my arms like that. It's not . . . passionate or sexy or anything – just very gentle and tender. Yes, I can see myself being like that with a baby.

> I can't help watching women with their babies. I'm curious. It's not the techniques of fixing a nappy or whatever, but how they touch their babies. Maybe that's a way of learning how to do it myself. I've never been around babies much. But now I can't help noticing them everywhere and I stare, I know I do. It's a kind of learning.

One way of enjoying closeness and getting in touch with your baby is to have some quiet time, a dream time, each day when you let thoughts form, shape and reshape themselves about the pregnancy, the baby and the birth. Ten or fifteen minutes is enough, though some women get to like this space in their otherwise busy lives so much that they stretch it to half an hour. They tell other people they are 'having a rest'. The point of this is not so much to rest physically but to make space for you and the baby together. It is the beginning of tuning in to the life that is to be, the first communication with your child, while it is still small enough to fit into the palm of your hand.

Some pregnant women are reluctant to do this in case they do not hold on to the pregnancy or there is something wrong with the baby or it dies. They feel that to allow themselves to bond with the baby while it is still inside them is dangerous. But even if this baby should not stay with you, even if there should be a miscarriage, for example, or if later you were to lose the child, there will have been someone with whom you have been in touch, whom you feel you have begun to know, a real little person to whom you have given yourself. The hardest thing of all is to grieve when you do not know exactly who you are grieving for, when the person you grieve for has no identity. Women whose babies have died at birth and who have not seen or held them often say this.

It may be that your partner, too, can make some quiet time to be with you and your developing baby. There is no need to talk. But once a couple have begun to enjoy this quiet space, other things happen. You may find that you stroke the gentle curve of your body in which the baby is cradled and talk to the baby. Do whatever you feel like doing.

> After each time of dreaming you may want to jot down your thoughts. They won't all be beautiful ones and it probably won't be great literature. Avoid censoring what comes. You are simply recording what is in your mind as you get more in touch with your feelings and in touch with your baby.

13

ON THE THRESHOLD
OF THE UNKNOWN

Every birth is an adventure. However many times a woman has done it before, she is setting out on a new experience which can bring unforeseen challenges.

> When you get to the last weeks take time to write in your notebook some of your impressions of this stage of your pregnancy – both emotional and physical. Describe the good feelings and the bad. Pick up any doubts or fears you have about the birth or afterwards. Write about your feelings for the baby in these weeks. You may want to write, too, about your hopes for your child and about how you want to be as a mother.
> It is easy to forget many of the thoughts and feelings you have now once the baby is born. Writing about them at this point can give you an important record of these final weeks of pregnancy.

For a woman having her first baby, the whole process may seem mysterious and awesome in its magnitude. She wonders how she will cope with pain, what contractions will feel like, how it will be when the baby's head slides out of her and pops like a pea out of its pod, whether she has any 'maternal instincts', and if, afterwards, she will ever be the same person again. Excitement, hope, curiosity and astonishment at the creative power expressing itself through her body are mingled with often only half-voiced fears and doubts about her own strength, ability and intrinsic worth.

Even when a woman already knows exactly what is involved in childbirth and has first-hand experience of being a mother, and thus is much more relaxed and pragmatic in her approach – she may still be not completely confident that she can cope with *this* labour and *this* baby.

A woman who already has a child may be much more tired than the first time round because she is busy nurturing her family and has little time to nurture herself. She often feels that this pregnancy is being crowded out – that she has no chance to concentrate on or enjoy it. It is as if this particular baby cannot be 'special' because she is swept up by everybody else's demands on her energy.

For one having her first baby who takes time off from work outside the home, on the other hand, these last weeks of pregnancy bring an unaccustomed space in her life and a feeling of leisure, though it will be short-lived. Even so, some women are beset with worries about getting behind with work and how they are going to cope with a baby and a job afterwards.

A woman on maternity leave discovers herself in a different world from that of her colleagues. As she becomes more and more baby-oriented, with prenatal visits, childbirth classes and getting everything ready, it may seem that 'real' life is going on at work without her. It can be frightening to change identity so swiftly and she may be anxious that she will never again be able to define herself as a capable working woman. The big question that seems to confront her is how she is going to 'fit' the baby into her life. In fact, whatever she does, her life is never going to be the same again!

By the end of pregnancy a woman longs to see and hold her baby and feels the mounting impatience and suspense of a child waiting for a birthday or Christmas to come and discover all she has been given. But even then eager anticipation is often mixed with anxiety and a feeling that she is not yet *ready*.

Whereas one woman thinks in terms of 'being delivered', another thinks of 'giving birth'. The very language used about birth reflects different attitudes to the whole process. When a woman is 'delivered' it implies that her role is passive. When she 'gives birth' she has an active role in creating new life. The first woman perceives her labour mainly as something which has to be endured for the sake of the baby, and the actions of the obstetrician who performs the delivery as of primary importance. The second sees her care-givers as peripheral to the main task of birth-giving, which, if everything turns out well, will be hers alone, and she looks forward to it as a fulfilling experience. Yet very much wanting birth to be natural and to bring satisfaction and fulfilment can impose its own stresses. If you are the sort of person who sets clear goals for yourself the last weeks are a time in which there is often a shadow of something like stage-fright. As the day when labour must begin draws nearer you may wonder if you will make a fool of yourself. You imagine yelling, swearing or pleading for pain-relieving drugs even if you have decided in advance that you do not want them. You may worry that you will not live up to some pre-set, frequently self-imposed standard and will disappoint your partner, your childbirth teacher – or yourself.

'He expects such a lot of me!' Sybil said. 'He's read all the books, religiously been to classes. I feel I've got to put on a star performance.'

'We've delayed having this baby until everything was just right – our careers, the house and so on,' Alison told me. 'We plan to have only one child and it matters a great deal to us that everything goes right – that I have natural childbirth, no drugs of any kind and breastfeed the baby immediately after birth.'

For her the script is all there. Now she feels it is up to her to play her part superbly well. No wonder that women under this kind of pressure are anxious that they will fail! Goal-oriented education which puts emphasis on success conditions us to approach childbirth as an athletic contest we are determined to win. And if it turns out that labour does not measure up to this pre-set goal, we then run the risk of feeling inadequate and guilty and being unable to enjoy the early weeks of motherhood.

Childbirth is not the kind of event in which you can dictate what happens or know in advance exactly how you are going to feel or what you are going to want to do. Like other life-processes which involve dramatic physical change and intense emotions, it cannot be planned in detail ahead of time – only *lived*. For it is, above all, an experience into which you bring not only your rational, planning self, but your whole being. When you make your birth plans it is important to remember this.

If you try to stick closely to some blueprint of how it 'ought' to be and how you 'should' behave, not only are you likely to be disappointed, but you can actually make it harder for yourself to live in the moment and let your feelings flow. The strength of the uterus, the whole powerful process of birth, is such an intense experience that if you are trying to control it you can feel as if you were desperately struggling to 'hold on to the reins', as if it were a runaway horse which you were trying to pull back.

Think through what you want, plan ahead, learn all you can, make your wishes clear to those who are giving you care, negotiate changes when routine practices do not match your priorities – but then, when labour starts, *give* yourself to the experience of birth.

Awkward positions

At the very end of the pregnancy you probably become very aware of different positions in which the baby lies – pressing against your ribs, or in the small of your back, bouncing against your vagina almost as if it were about to fall out, or leaning against your bladder. These physical changes of late pregnancy, which result from the baby dropping lower and settling itself into a position for birth, may mean that you feel almost full to bursting, and there is hardly a moment when you are not conscious of the imminent arrival of your baby.

By 36 weeks many babies, especially in first pregnancies, have engaged in the pelvis in a position ready for birth. Others have not. They are still changing position. This is likely if it is your second baby and still more usual if you have had two or three babies before, because the uterus will have stretched, so the baby is not such a tight fit. Sometimes a baby is lying transverse – right across the uterus, with the bottom on one side and the head on the other. You may be worried, because when a baby is transverse during labour it gets stuck and has to be delivered by Caesarean section. But in practice this rarely happens, because the baby's head is the heaviest part and by the time labour starts the baby will nearly always have rolled over with its head down in the cervix. The official name for all this is 'unstable lie', and it sounds ominous. In fact, all it means is that the baby is not fixed in one position or another.

Coaxing a breech to a vertex

Most babies are head down in the uterus by some time during the seventh month. Others remain stubbornly bottom down, though when they have not yet engaged in the pelvis they can still move fairly freely into different positions. But when a baby engages as a breech and gets more or less fixed in the pelvis it is not going to disengage and somersault over unless you, or your doctor, take active steps to change the position. And even then it may fit the available space in your pelvis more comfortably sitting up, so may turn back again.

Both ends of the baby have to be born anyway, of course, but the head dilates the opening better than the buttocks, and the problem with a breech is that if the body is born but there is still not enough room for the biggest part, the head, there can be delay at delivery, during which the baby can be short of oxygen. That is why breech babies are often delivered by 'forceps on the after-coming head' or by Caesarean section.

If your baby has started to go down into the pelvis as a breech there are ways you may be able to persuade it to turn. Wait until this point is reached, or the baby may simply go back again immediately. Being inside the pelvis restricts movement.

First feel with your fingers exactly how your baby is lying. You can get help with this from your doctor or midwife. With a breech baby you are probably familiar with the feeling of the head like a coconut against your midriff. Leg movements occur in the lower part of your abdomen, unless the baby is lying with its feet by its shoulders, in which case it is splinted by its own legs and does not move much at all.

To coax the baby to change position you first need to tip it out of the bony cradle of your pelvis. Choose a time during the day: there is no point in doing it and lying down afterwards, because the baby may then turn back. Start by lying with your bottom high, head down, for 20 to 30 minutes. A large, firm bean-bag, or even two piled one on the other, will allow you to be reasonably comfortable in this odd position. Make a deep dip for your tummy and lie on your front. The baby's back and head are its heaviest parts and since you want the head down and the back forward for it to be in the best position, it is good for you to be on your front rather than your back, and to reduce the pressure against your abdomen. You can probably help this by slightly bending your knees, so that your bottom is even higher. A divan bed and plenty of pillows, arranged so that you kneel up on the side or end of the bed, with your head on a pillow on the floor, can also be used. You may have other furniture which you can adapt for this purpose.

Once you have been lying in this position for some time the baby will tip free of the pelvis and may start to move. Keep your head down and bottom up, and check with your hands the position of the head. Can you still feel it pressing against your diaphragm? It may, of course, stay that way. But often the baby will somersault over and suddenly the big, round lump in your middle is gone, and instead you can feel smaller lumps under your ribs, often to one side only – the baby's feet. If this happens, someone should help you get up (you may feel a bit dizzy), and you then keep standing and moving about for the next hour or so – perhaps go for a long walk – to see if you can fix the baby in your pelvis head down.

When a doctor turns a baby it is called 'external version'. You adopt a head-down position for 20 minutes, and the doctor then grasps the head and buttocks through your abdomen and turns the baby, usually in the direction of its nose. (It should be done carefully, or the placenta can be pulled away from its moorings.) This procedure is preferable to Caesarean section, but many doctors no longer know how to do it.

Coaxing a posterior to anterior

What if your baby is head down, but with its limbs to the front? You can tell if this is so because you feel all the movement at the front, there is a saucer-shaped dip by your navel, which is the space between the arms and legs, and the hard back of the baby is pressing against your sacrum (the bone where your pelvis joins your spine) so you probably have back-ache – though bad posture can cause this too, so you cannot be certain just from this. When the baby is anterior a woman's navel usually sticks out like a button in the last few weeks. When the baby is posterior, it still looks like an ordinary navel.

Doctors do not attempt to turn posteriors to anteriors, except inter-nally with forceps or manually just before delivery. But traditionally midwives have coaxed babies round with massage in some peasant cultures, and there is no reason why you should not have a go at this yourself. If you have a small pelvic inlet, the baby may need to enter it in a posterior position, but can turn round, sometimes with a bit of persuasion, into a better anterior position for birth.

Wait until the head has negotiated the pelvic inlet, because the baby will be moving around all over the place before then anyway. Moreover, if you can persuade the baby to turn round, it will help to fix the head in the new position if it is inside the pelvis like an egg in an eggcup.

To change an anterior to a posterior, wait until your baby is awake and moving. In this way the baby may help you. Now get on all fours with your tummy hanging down. First feel how your baby is lying. Can you find the back? It may be right round to the back and difficult to feel at all. It is often on your right-hand side, but tilted round towards your back. Sometimes it is in a similar position on your left. See if you can get the palm of your hand around it. Rock your pelvis up and down a bit. Then, once you can feel the back, grasp it firmly, as if it were a kitten you were trying to slide along the sofa so you could sit down, and little by little press and stroke it round towards the front with a deep scooping movement, every now and again rocking your pelvis. Because the back is heavier than the limbs, there may be a point at which it simply falls forward. And that's it!

Now either keep upright for an hour or so or, if you do lie down, avoid lying on your back, or the baby may turn round again immediately.

Sometimes a baby will not turn, but does move from an extended position to curl up into a ball, and that is an improvement too.[1] Sometimes, even if you manage to turn the baby successfully, it goes back again. You may need to repeat the manoeuvre at intervals before the baby fixes as anterior. Some babies will not turn, and then you will have to wait for strong contractions in labour to press the baby into a more compact ball and rotate it into a good position. If given enough time, seven out of ten babies rotate to the anterior during labour.

One disconcerting thing about prenatal examinations is that a woman is expected to lie on her back for her abdomen to be palpated. The result is that her baby may roll round to a posterior position. This is why your doctor may find the baby is posterior, whereas when you are lying on your side, turned over towards your front, on all fours or standing, you may notice that the smooth, firm sweep of the back is towards your front, which means the baby must be anterior. This is a good reason for deciding to adopt upright, forward-leaning and all-fours positions in labour.

Once you are in the 36th week of your pregnancy note down any observations you have about your baby's position and any changes in it. Get help from your doctor or midwife if you are uncertain. If you decide to try either of these ways of coaxing the baby to a different position, record what happened.

Changes in your body

The physical changes of pregnancy are so powerful, and in the last few weeks so inescapable, that for many women it seems as if they are on the edge of a new state of being, as this familiar body starts to open in order to push out into the world another living creature.

Once the baby has dipped into the pelvis it often feels to the pregnant woman as if her insides are being slowly but inexorably sucked downwards; that not just the baby, but everything is slipping lower, ready to drop out. When the baby has engaged, the head presses so low that it feels like a coconut swinging between your legs. You may have a fantasy of waters bursting and everything happening in the middle of the local supermarket.

Physical sensations experienced during the last weeks of pregnancy are not so much painful as odd. You may not be able to get completely comfortable in any position. At times it feels as if you are lumbering around like a tank. On good days it is more as if you were a ship in full sail.

There are advantages – even some pleasures – in occupying a larger space than usual. Though it is rarely talked about, the magnitude and splendour of advanced pregnancy may bring with it a sense of power. The woman moves with the great globe of her uterus pressing under her ribcage and down against the muscles slung across the base of her hip-bones, the skin stretched taut over her abdomen, a huge curved dome, with the baby safely inside, rolling and kicking beneath it like a dolphin playing. Other people move away, giving her space. They may be considerate and caring, awed, or perhaps just fearful that labour will start and they will have to deliver the baby.

If you already have children, they react to your changed shape very differently from adults. They play on the bump, lean against and poke it and climb and crawl over it. They sit or lie on it, knock, press and prod it. They may talk to the little creature inside. The baby is already part of the family!

The sheer weight carried around in the last weeks of pregnancy tends to make a woman very tired at the end of the day and ready for an early bed. At a rough guess there are 7 to 9 pounds (3 to 4 kilograms) of baby, $1\frac{1}{2}$ to 2 pounds ($\frac{3}{4}$ to 1 kilo) of placenta, $1\frac{1}{2}$ to 2 pounds ($\frac{3}{4}$ to 1 kilo) of amniotic fluid, 2 pounds (1 kilo) of uterus, a pound ($\frac{1}{2}$ kilo) or more of extra breast tissue, 2 pounds (1 kilo) of extra blood, 2 to $2\frac{1}{2}$ pounds (around a kilo) of water in the tissues and about 8 to 9 pounds ($3\frac{1}{2}$ to 4 kilos) of personal body fat: total – 25 to 30 pounds ($11\frac{1}{2}$ to $13\frac{1}{2}$ kilos).

When you go to bed it may be hard to find a position in which you can easily drop off to sleep. You can shift pillows around to support a leg, cradle the bump or press against an aching back. Even so, once off to sleep you may wake to discover that the baby is sky-diving against your bladder, and there are frequent trips to the lavatory. Some babies move so much, even in the last weeks of pregnancy when they must be short of space, that they wake their mothers constantly with a foot protruding under the ribs or a belly-roll like a tidal wave.

Pressure against the pelvic floor muscles which support bladder, rectum and uterus from underneath is so intense at this stage that they may be stretched. When you cough, sneeze or laugh you may wet your pants. Hormones released into the bloodstream have softened and loosened your body for birth, but made daily life more complicated.

This softening has its positive aspect, too, for it brings a sense of physical succulence and richness. The accordion-like folds of the vagina are thick and full now, ready to open out as the baby's head presses through. The cervix is being drawn up into the main body of the uterus and is also softening like ripe, squashy fruit about to ooze its juice. The breasts are veined and full, ready to give thick, creamy colostrom. The uterus is tightening intermittently as if preparing for its task in labour. This may happen so often, and contractions become so strong and regular near term, that you think you must be in labour, though in fact it is just an energetic rehearsal.

Labour can start, in fact, in several different ways. You may notice you are having contractions which become stronger, longer and closer together over a period of some two hours. Anything less than this and it is best not to decide you are in labour. You may be aware that the mucus plug has come out and that you have passed a pink 'show' – much like the very start of a period – but this can happen a couple of weeks before you actually begin labour. Or your waters may leak or break in a rush. And this again may occur before you feel any contractions, though they usually start within five to eight hours.

Premature rupture of the membranes

If the waters leak before labour starts and the baby, though viable, would be very premature, doctors are agreed that they should try to keep the pregnancy going as long as possible. Steroids may be given to the mother in order to help the baby's lungs to mature and so avoid the respiratory distress syndrome common in very pre-term babies. (However, it is possible that steroids may make the baby less able to resist infection after birth.) If membranes rupture when the baby would be premature, but not dangerously so, doctors disagree about what should be done. Some admit the mother to hospital for rest in bed and to wait and see. Some believe in performing amniocentesis to assess the maturity of the baby's lungs, and if the signs are good will then induce labour.

When membranes rupture near term, many doctors believe that labour should be induced if it does not start spontaneously in 24 hours, or 12 hours, or whatever is the particular time limit they impose, because they are concerned that pelvic infection or infection of the baby may result. So a woman is usually told to go into hospital immediately, is put to bed, and lies around hoping against hope that contractions will begin.

This is not a good way to start a labour. It introduces stress and anxiety because something seems to be going wrong, and even though you are feeling completely healthy you are straight away transformed into a sick person.

The possibility of premature rupture of the membranes is one of the insidious worries in some pregnant women's minds in those last weeks of pregnancy. They are often told by their childbirth teacher and by the doctor that if there is any leaking of water they must take immediate action and go to hospital because of the risk of infection. Infection, however, is sometimes the *cause* rather than the consequence of premature rupture of the membranes, and it seems to start in the underlying layer of membranes, not in the outside layer.[2]

The usual prophylactic treatment when membranes rupture prematurely consists of antibiotics and, after some hours of hopeful anticipation, induction of labour. Occasionally membranes seal up again spontaneously after an initial leak. This sometimes happens if the leak was in the hind-waters, above the baby's chin, rather than in the fore-waters which form a bubble below the head. No one knows how it is that membranes can seal over again. But once you have started to lose water it usually goes on flowing.

If induction is proposed there are several things to discuss with your obstetrician. There is no need to take it for granted that from now on everything is abnormal and the whole thing must be treated as a medical crisis.

It would be useful to know whether or not your cervix is ripe and partially effaced (drawn up into the uterus). There may be evidence of this already in your records so it may not entail having another vaginal examination. If the cervix is not ripe, labour which is started artificially is likely to last longer than spontaneous labour and there is an increased chance of it ending in a Caesarean section.[3] On the other hand, it is important to bear in mind that when the interval between rupture of the membranes and delivery exceeds 24 hours, vaginal examinations increase the risk of infection. A Dutch study reveals, however, that infection is no more likely *when no vaginal examinations are performed*.[4] Occasionally the membranes seal themselves over again and a woman does not go into labour for some days, the membranes rupturing anew once labour has started.

There is a strong case to be made, therefore, for waiting expectantly, having no vaginal examinations, and taking your temperature every four hours to check if there is any rise which could indicate that you have an infection. It is also a good idea to smell the amniotic fluid every time you change your pad, since the very first sign of infection is an unpleasant odour. A prophylactic course of antibiotics will further reduce the chances of developing an infection. Provided that you do not become feverish and that the water remains clear and odourless, there is no good case to be made for induction of labour. The membranes may have ruptured early merely because there was a weak spot in them, and this sometimes seems to happen at the end of a pregnancy in which there was amniocentesis.

Leaking of the waters is not, after all, such a bad way to start labour. You have warning that something is about to happen soon and can make preparations. Nor, if labour starts naturally, does it mean that it is likely to be longer, more arduous or more painful, though doctors are trained to treat premature rupture of the membranes as an abnormality and often want to intervene.

Thinking ahead to how you would want to cope if this happened can help you retain your own autonomy, share in decision-making with your doctor and stay calm, relaxed and looking forward to your labour.

The Way Birth Is

14

THE JOURNEY THROUGH LABOUR

Before you set out on an unfamiliar journey it helps to have a rough idea of the territory you are going to cover, challenges you may meet on your way and the steps you can take to cope effectively with them. Though each labour is different, there is a common unfolding pattern to childbirth, and it is important to be aware of this so that you are prepared for the various phases and are not shocked by sudden changes in the feelings you are experiencing. It is vital for your birth companion to understand these things too, if he or she is to give you strong and confident support.

Each birth is in some ways like a theatrical production. There is a lead-in which is rather like a prologue, a first scene which serves to introduce the plot and characters, increased concentration and involvement in the action as the plot thickens, often intervals when nothing much seems to be happening and you can take a break, and a build-up of excitement to the grand finale – the birth of your baby.

Though the medical view of labour is that it is divided into three stages, the first stage being dilatation of the cervix, the second expulsion of the infant and the third delivery of the placenta – like a three-act play – you may experience many phases within the first and second 'acts' which have different, and even contrasting, moods and kinds of action for which you need to be prepared.

However enthusiastically you start out on labour, there are often times when morale drops and you feel tired and irritable, times when you feel bewildered and anxious about what is going to happen next and occasions when there is fear, doubt, frustration or insecurity. Learning how to deal with these negative elements is important if you are to be well rehearsed for your part in the drama of birth.

The schematic outline of labour presented on the following pages is divided into columns which suggest what might be happening in your body, how you may feel, what you can do to help yourself, and how your birth companion can best give support at each stage. There are no rules to be followed, but the outline can give you an indication of how birth is for other women, so that you can learn from their experiences.

The Pattern of Labour

PHASE	PHYSICAL SIGNS	HOW YOU MAY FEEL	HOW YOU CAN HELP YOURSELF	WHAT BIRTH COMPANION CAN DO TO HELP
Pre-labour – the last few days of pregnancy	Some thinning out (effacement), ripening and possible dilatation of cervix.	Anticipation. Exhilaration.	Prepare everything needed for birth.	Make sure you can be reached easily at all times.
	Increased and stronger Braxton-Hicks contractions.	Some self-doubt likely: am I going to be able to cope?	Get regular rest and sleep. Take exercise.	Take over some household tasks.
	Baby's head may engage in pelvis.	Surge of energy – 'nesting'.	Gentle massage of nipples will help cervix ripen.	Give emotional support.
	May have 'show' – like beginning of period.*			If woman likes it, stroke and play with one nipple at a time to help ripening of cervix.
	May have loose bowel motions.			
	May have low backache.			
Early first stage	Cervix is being drawn up and thinned out.	Excited. Confident.	Have light meal – e.g., soup, omelette, bread and honey, banana, grapes.	If things start slowly, have meal together in relaxing setting (e.g., in garden), or picnic in country, go out to restaurant or invite friends in.
	1–5 cm dilatation. 'Show' if have not had it before.*		Relax in bath.	
	Contractions get longer, stronger and are at regular intervals, 5 minutes or more apart. They may be like indigestion, cramps, period pains or band of elastic pulling in round lower abdomen.		Alternate rest and activity if daytime. Get some sleep if night time or if you need it.	Choose distracting activity together – e.g., watch film, do light gardening or cooking, invite friends round or go out and visit friends, play Scrabble or cards, walk in country.
			Do some cooking which takes a long time – e.g., bread, meringues, slow casserole.	

* If steady bleeding occurs ring doctor.

Waters may break with slow leak, or pop so that water streams out.		Empty bladder every 1½ hours. If not sure that this is labour, try completely different activity – e.g.. if in bed, get up and do something; if up, have rest or watch TV. If contractions are big enough not to be able to talk through them, start slow, full breathing. Relax.	Help her relax. Stay calm, confident, loving. Make sure any phone numbers needed are handy, and if using car there is petrol in tank. Help with household tasks. Rub her back or stroke her abdomen.
Late first stage	5–8 cm dilatation. Contractions get stronger, longer, closer together, till every 2–3 minutes and lasting 60 seconds or more. Waters may go.	General sense of everything getting faster and more intense. Feel you want to concentrate on labour. Get more serious. May become apprehensive, discouraged, impatient, irritated. May feel tired. May feel trapped. May vomit.	Go to hospital or birth room if not already there. Discuss birth plan with midwife. Focus concentration during contractions. Drop shoulders and relax as each one starts. Welcome each contraction with slow breath out. Breathe more lightly if you need to over peak of contraction. Give long breath out as contraction finishes. Doze between contractions and relax completely.
			Help her relax. Use touch, stroking, firm holding, or massage. Put cold cloth on her forehead between contractions. Rest warm cloth or hot water bottle against lower abdomen, between thighs, over lower back. Offer iced water and ice-chips. Breathe with her if this helps. For backache: use strong counter-pressure, ice wrapped in cloth, or hot towel. Help her change position to leaning forward.

Late first stage

PHASE	PHYSICAL SIGNS	HOW YOU MAY FEEL	HOW YOU CAN HELP YOURSELF	WHAT BIRTH COMPANION CAN DO TO HELP
Late first stage			Use aerosol water-spray or small plant spray to freshen up.	Help her move and walk around.
			Move around and change position as often as wished.	
			Empty bladder every 1½ hours.	
			Suck ice-chips, sip liquid or suck on sponge.	
			For backache, hands and knees position, walking, side-lying, kneeling or sitting forward.	
Transition: bridge between first and second stages	8–10 cm dilated.	As if tossed in a storm at sea.	Welcome each contraction with a long, slow breath out. Then breathe as lightly and quickly as you want to.	Stay with her. You are her anchor in a stormy sea.
	Contractions powerful, every 1½–2 minutes and lasting 90 seconds, or almost continuous.	Restless, increased irritability, sense of time lost.		Remind her that transition, though intense, is short.
	Some contractions may have double peaks.	May not want to be touched.	Concentrate on one contraction at a time. That particular one will never come back again.	Give her information. Remind her of baby, signs of progress, 'not long now'.
	Concentrated pain around cervix as final tissue is pulled up over baby's head	May be forgetful and even forget you are having a baby.	Relax buttocks and pelvic floor like heavy hammock.	Encourage and reassure her. Speak simply and clearly.

and baby is pressed down through cervix.	Find it difficult to relax completely and keep breathing rhythms.	Be responsive to her mood. Breathe with her if this helps.
Cramp in legs.	May want to give up.	Maintain peaceful atmosphere.
Feel hot – then cold – then hot.	May be frightened because everything is over-whelming.	Give hot water bottle between legs, at feet, in small of back, or she may prefer ice in towel for back pain.
Cold feet.	May feel urge to push.	
Drowsiness.	May fall asleep between contractions.	Help her change position. She may get stuck and uncomfortable in one position.
Shaking.		
Flushed face.		She may appreciate massage, stroking, firm holding, having her back rubbed. If she is shaking, firm massage of inner thighs may help. Use whole palm of each hand, fingers pointing down, and massage from tops of inside legs to knees, stroking back lightly over tops of legs, keeping continuous rhythmic movement.
Hiccups, catch in throat, belching, involuntarily holding breath, grunting, groaning on breath out at end of contraction – all signs of pushing urge.	Walk around, change position for comfort.	
	Use any rest times for complete relaxation.	
Waters may go if they have not gone before.	Blow out if feel urge to push and attendant says not to push yet.	Offer sips of iced water and ice-chips. Vaseline or lip salve for lips.
May begin to feel pressure against rectum.		She may like a sponge-down with cool or hot water.

The Pattern of Labour

PHASE	PHYSICAL SIGNS	HOW YOU MAY FEEL	HOW YOU CAN HELP YOURSELF	WHAT BIRTH COMPANION CAN DO TO HELP
'Rest and be thankful' interval	Full dilatation. Contractions often become weak or fade away for about 20 minutes, sometimes longer.	Sense of peace. Anxiety because no contractions felt if told to start pushing.	Rest. Close eyes. Enjoy lull.	Relax. Wait patiently. Brush her hair back from her face, offer cologne, and freshen her up for pushing. Reassure her that all is well. Give encouragement. Play soft, relaxing music. A shower may feel good.
Second stage	Urge to push gets stronger as the baby comes lower. Contractions may be further apart. Degree and timing of pushing urge may vary with each contraction. 1–4 urges, coming in waves, during each contraction. A little blood may appear when pushing; may have small bowel movement.	Cheerful, excited. Amazed at power of pushing urge, as if you are *being* pushed rather than pushing. May feel very tired and doze between contractions. Completely absorbed in what you are doing and not concerned about surroundings. Renewed determination as you see and feel baby's	Right time to push is when *you* want to; you should push only as and when your body tells you to: hold breath only as long as you need to. Do whatever you feel like doing. Change position often for comfort; try kneeling, crouching, squatting, on all fours, supported standing squat.	Encourage her by saying 'Open up' and 'Good' – *not* 'Push' – with contractions. Rest hot cloth over anus and perineum if she finds it helps her relax pelvic floor muscles. Help her change position so that upper part of body is well raised. Position in which she is most comfortable is right.

Feels as if grapefruit in anus – then this changes to head. Burst of energy. Feeling of heat builds up until it is like 'ring of fire' around baby's head.

Crowning.

Birth of baby's head – then whole body slips out.

Relax perineum, buttocks, legs.

Touch top of baby's head before it is born.

Breathe out baby.

Interest turns to baby.

Put hands down to feel whole head when it has slid out.

Feel cannot stretch any more without popping.

Reach out arms for baby and do whatever comes naturally.

Relief – astonishment – joy – gratitude – ecstasy.

Let feelings flow.

If progress is slow, help her squat. Support her physically in different positions: standing, kneeling, or sitting behind her so that her back is supported.

Sponge her with cold water between contractions; offer ice-chips.

Remind her to open eyes to see birth.

Tell her when head can be seen.

If she is using delivery mirror, adjust its angle as necessary so that she can see her perineum.

As head is about to crown, breathe with her, mouth open, to enable head to be born gently.

Watch birth.

Welcome baby! Let feelings flow. Kiss, embrace, stroke, hold each other – whatever comes spontaneously.

PHASE	PHYSICAL SIGNS	HOW YOU MAY FEEL	HOW YOU CAN HELP YOURSELF	WHAT BIRTH COMPANION CAN DO TO HELP
Third stage	Delivery of placenta and membranes in 45 minutes or so. In 5 minutes if injection given to stimulate uterus. Contractions milder, further apart. Bleeding should only be about ½ pint. Maybe uncontrolled shaking.	Completely engrossed in baby, or may need time to come to terms with power of experience, recover from shock and reality of birth. Excited, tired.	Express love, triumph, wonder, feelings that well up. Relax, hold and enjoy baby. Watch for when baby opens eyes. Push to expel placenta; ask to see it if interested.	Hold and enjoy baby. Help her get baby on to breast when he/she begins to root for nipple. Put warm blanket over mother and baby. Hold in arms.

Labour rehearsal

In the last 6 weeks of pregnancy it is useful to make time for a talk with your future birth companion about his or her role in helping you. This may be your partner, a family member or a friend. Whoever it is, they should understand the kind of preparation you have been making for labour and, if possible, have attended at least some classes with you. It is important that they are confident and calm, and this is made easier if they understand what is happening, what you are trying to do, and how they can help.

The chart in the last few pages gives you information about what happens, how you might feel and how your labour companion can help you. Select from it some phases in labour and first talk about and then act through what you might do and the help you would want in these circumstances.

To simulate a contraction, your partner can take hold of a little flesh from your inside thigh (not over a varicose vein) and squeeze it gradually tighter and tighter over a period of 30 seconds or so, then gradually release it for another 30 seconds. Breathe and relax into it. Start with some fairly easy 'contractions' and move on to difficult ones. You may find they make you feel angry, frustrated, irritable, trapped – all emotions which may flood through you in labour too. How can you handle the next contraction better? What do you want your helper to do? (In labour, fortunately, your companion will have both hands free and will not have to act the part of the uterus too!)

Include in your rehearsal different ways in which you might start labour. Imagine one that starts slowly, one that begins with the waters breaking, or with contractions only two minutes apart. Imagine having a short, sharp labour; a long-drawn-out, tiring, backache labour; an induced labour; even a surprise birth without anyone else there to help – and so on. Talk about how you feel and what your needs are. You might want to say, for example, 'It would have been better if you had massaged me *here*,' or 'I wanted to be quite quiet.'

It may help to say, 'I need from you . . .' (and finish the sentence by telling your helper what is most important for you). There are other phrases which may be useful too: 'I am afraid that . . .'; 'I hope . . .'; 'I want you to give me . . .'

Your support person will approach the birth with expectations and doubts of their own. It can be useful to bring these out into the open also and to discuss them. Here are some phrases that may help to express these: 'I know that . . .'; 'I'm not sure that . . .'; 'I shall be glad if . . .'

There are, of course, many other ways in which you could talk about feelings and I do not mean this to be a formal exercise. But some discussion like this can help you get on the same wavelength.

As you do this, include as much practical action as you can. For example, if you want to go to the lavatory, do you want your birth companion with you? If so, what would you like them to do: hold your shoulders, your feet, your hands – or just be there? If you have a shower, do you want your birth companion to stay with you? (If so, in hospital a man should bring bathing trunks.) Does it help to be held? Is it important to maintain eye contact? You have cramp in your leg; what do you want done about this? You are thirsty, what do you want? You have slipped too low against the pillows and want them more upright. You are over-breathing or tensing up your legs. How can most effective help be given?

You may find that labour is very different from what you expected and that some things you practised beforehand are irrelevant. The point of these rehearsals is that you make a close working partnership so that, whatever happens, your birth companion is sensitively responsive to your moods and you are intimately in touch.

HAPPY BIRTHDAY!

15

DEALING WITH PAIN

A central issue for many women is how they are going to cope with pain. Most women get some pain in labour, but find it manageable. Some, however, have more than they can handle without help. It helps to understand *why* you are experiencing pain. Then you can make plans about how to deal with it. Pain is most likely in the following situations:

- If the baby is a very tight fit for the woman's pelvis – cephalo-pelvic disproportion (CPD). The baby's head is not hard bone all over. The skull bones are in sections which are pressed towards and can even slide over each other. Since the uterus squeezes the baby's head, its largest part, rather as if it were a ripe grapefruit, to fit the outlet available, a woman with small bones can often bear a large baby, but the process may be painful.

- If the woman's uterus is short of oxygen. Though some researchers do not accept that this is a cause of pain, it is possible that cramp-like discomfort occurs when the uterus is not getting enough oxygen. Any muscle aches when insufficiently oxygenated. If there is not enough time for the uterus to become oxygenated between contractions, they may hurt a great deal. Breathing slowly and fully between contractions, and at the beginning and end of each, oxygenates the blood and this oxygen is carried to the uterus.

- If the woman's cervix is slow to open. The baby's head presses through the cervix as if a tight roll-neck sweater was being pulled over it.[1] The cervix is very flexible and can open up more and more, given time, but it can be tough going.

- If the baby is in an awkward position. Though breech (bottom first) labours are often not especially painful, if the baby is head down but lying with its back towards the woman's own back, the crown does not fit over the cervix, and the back of the head, the *occiput*, presses into the small of the back, causing backache. Labour with a baby in an occipito-posterior position like this may be painful and tiring because it can take a long time for the contractions to turn the baby's head into the correct anterior position.

- If the uterus is not working efficiently. Contractions are huge and painful, but because there is incoordinate uterine action the cervix does not dilate. No one knows why this happens, but sometimes it is because the baby is lying awkwardly.

- If labour is very long (24 hours or more) and the woman is suffering from lack of sleep. It can be difficult to cope with a normal 8- to 12-hour labour if you have had inadequate sleep the night before. Labour demands energy and stamina. This is why it is important to be well rested when you start. If you are having your baby in hospital, avoid going in too soon. Many more women go in too early than too late. They are at risk of having labour accelerated with oxytocin, and a whole range of other interventions, simply because they have gone to hospital before they needed to.

How we feel about what is happening in our bodies is just as important as what is occurring physiologically. Negative feelings can intrude on childbirth and make it more painful in these situations:

- If a woman is afraid, very anxious, angry or frustrated, demanding a great deal of herself and struggling to keep control of a labour that she finds confusing and muddled. Emotions can help or hinder labour and reduce or increase the perception of pain.

- If a woman is sure that labour is going to be excruciatingly painful, she may get in such a state of tension that even an ordinary touch hurts. It is an unfailing recipe for a painful labour. Grantly Dick-Read, who introduced the concept of natural childbirth, taught that ignorance produces fear, which leads to tension, which creates pain. Yet knowing what is happening to you and what other people are doing to help – even knowing how to help yourself – though important, may not be enough. Any emotions which prevent you feeling free and acting spontaneously can sharpen pain and make it intolerable. This is why it is important to think in advance about emotional aspects of birth.

- If a woman is in the hands of people she does not like or trust. The environment for birth has a great deal to do with the amount of pain she feels. When she feels trapped in a situation in which she is controlled by others, she cannot do simple, easy things to handle discomfort, and pain feels more severe.

- If a woman has not allowed herself to believe that labour might be painful, any pain experienced can be overwhelming. Pain is a normal part of most labours. It usually occurs only during contractions, and for much of the time is slight at the beginning and end of contractions, but strong as they reach their peak. Each contraction is followed by a rest period of about five minutes early in labour, one minute or less as she approaches full dilatation of the cervix. Many women have no pain at all as they are pushing the baby out, though the feeling of the head like a grapefruit against the anus and then pressing through the vagina is often alarming. If you hope to have your baby without drugs it is important to be able to accept the idea of pain.

- If a woman has not learnt and *practised* ways of handling pain herself. She is then left at the receiving end of powerful sensations she can do nothing about. Breathing, relaxation, changes of posture, movement, massage, focused concentration, visualization (picturing what is happening inside your body), meditation, self-hypnosis, acupuncture and acupressure, hypnosis – all these can help you handle pain in a constructive way.

If you look back over the list you will see there is action you can take about most of the causes of pain. So go through them one by one and work out ways in which you can prepare yourself. You may decide, for example, that in case the baby is posterior you need to know and practise in advance positions, movements and massage for dealing with backache labour. Since it is often people closest to a woman who are anxious that she should get into hospital once labour seems to have started, you can discuss with your partner the disadvantages of going in too soon and plan things you could do together early in labour. You may decide that you need to set aside more time to rehearse labour and ways in which you can handle pain, and arrange a regular half-hour each day to do so in future. If you have been avoiding thinking about pain, the time has probably come to talk about it with some women who have had babies recently and find out exactly how they felt and what helped them most. You can also think back to the last time you had a pain – period pains are a good example – or, if it is not your first baby, how it felt in your previous labour – and note what helped you cope best, or things that in retrospect you wish you had done. As you watch TV, read or sew, you can prepare for the sensation of the baby's head on your perineum by sitting on the floor with your back straight against a wall, the soles of your feet together near your buttocks, and feeling your pelvis wide open. Be aware of the space in your vagina and imagine the weight of the baby's head like a coconut ready to drop. Or try squatting, feet well apart and back rounded as you hold on to furniture, and visualize yourself completely open.

Pain-relieving drugs

In obstetrically directed birth the doctor decides when and if drugs are necessary in order to control pain, and the patient does not have the freedom to cope with pain in any way she wishes. Pain is reduced or eradicated by something done *to* her rather than something she does for herself, and drugs are used as a first, rather than a last, resort.

When powerful pain-relieving drugs are employed a woman becomes dependent on her care-givers for their administration and topping-up, for constant monitoring of the condition of herself and the baby, and other procedures which may be ordered as a consequence of drug use. The more effective the medication, the more other interventions a woman may have. Strong drugs can interfere with the action of the uterus and slow down labour, so measures may be taken to stimulate the uterus. This may entail further intervention to monitor the fetal heart rate and the use of other drugs which act as antidotes to those given for pain relief. If a woman cannot feel contractions, decisions may be taken to accelerate labour or to lift the baby out by forceps.

Analgesics (pain-relieving drugs) and anaesthetics (pain-eradicating drugs) are often advised by obstetricians because it enables them to have more control over the birth process. One obstetrician has explained that having anaesthesia in labour is like having local anaesthetic for a dental filling, and, 'just as a pain-free non-squirming relaxed patient enabled dentists to perform their task smoothly, so did an epidural give rise to a relaxed, manageable and accessible mother'.[2]

On the other hand, drugs for pain relief have a definite place in childbirth – especially when there are deviations from the normal and a woman is in severe pain. There is no need for any woman to 'prove' her womanhood by labouring without drugs when she is experiencing more pain than she is prepared to cope with. It is often claimed that supporters of 'natural childbirth' do not approve of any drugs. The founding father of the natural childbirth movement, Grantly Dick-Read, expressed a very different point of view when he said: 'To tolerate suffering when it can be relieved is no less brutal than to insist on suffering when it is not present . . . The administration of anaesthetics and analgesics should have definite indication in obstetrics as it has in every branch of medicine or surgery.' [3]

As you consider the benefits and hazards of different kinds of anaesthesia and discuss them with your doctor and midwife, these are some of the things you can ask:

How is it given?

What effect will it have on me in the lowest dose available . . . in the highest dose available?

What effect might it have on the progress of labour? Does this depend on the time when it is given . . . the dosage?

What effect is it likely to have on the baby? Is this dependent on timing and dosage? If so, how?

Are any long-term side-effects experienced by the mother? If so what are these?

Could there be long-term side-effects for the baby? If so what are these?

What alternatives are available? Is this method of pain relief available at any time in the 24 hours? Can it be given so that, if I wish, its effect wears off by the time the second stage starts?

Is there a higher incidence of forceps delivery with this kind of anaesthesia?

What do you see as the main advantages of this kind of pain relief . . . main disadvantages?

You will obviously not want to ask all these questions at one time and the answers you get will probably make some of them unnecessary. But they are useful questions to keep in the back of your mind during any discussion about drugs.

Drugs used in labour

Sedatives (e.g., barbiturates, chloral) may be offered early in labour. They cause drowsiness and if the latent phase is long may enable you to get some sleep. A disadvantage is that they often lead to disorientation and once the active phase starts a woman may be struggling to cope with contractions which prove overwhelming, since each time she is roused from heavy sleep. Sedatives should not be given within four hours of delivery as they depress the baby's respiration.

Antihistamines (e.g., Phenergan) and *tranquillizers* (e.g., Largactil, Sparine, Vallergan, Valium) are used to calm the mother. Tranquillizers reduce anxiety and some, like antihistamines, are used to treat nausea and vomiting as well. One disadvantage is that they may make the woman feel drunk and out of control. They can also produce dizziness and blurred vision. They should not be given within four hours of delivery because they cause respiratory depression and poor muscle tone in the newborn and lead to feeding difficulties.

They may be used alone or in combination with narcotics (see below).

Narcotics (e.g., Demerol [in the USA] or pethidine [in Britain], morphine, mepezidine – a morphine derivative – and, in some countries, heroin) may be offered once dilatation of the cervix is progressing well. The dose should be related to the woman's weight. They have the effect of muffling pain, but also cause confusion and can make a woman feel powerless to cope actively with labour. Sometimes there are vivid dreams or hallucinations. The effects of these drugs last three to four hours. When given too soon they stop dilatation. But since they pass through the placenta and into the baby's bloodstream, they should not be given within four hours of delivery. Break-down products build up in the baby, who thus suffers more from the central nervous system depressant effects of the drugs than the mother, and the baby's breathing is depressed for longer than pain relief works for the mother. An antidote can be injected into her, or into the baby after birth if breathing is slow to start. It is not known if this has any long-term effects on the baby.

Hypnotics may also be used in combination with narcotics. They sedate the mother and cause amnesia – i.e., they do not eradicate pain, but destroy the memory of it. The best known, Scopolamine, often causes extreme restlessness and confusion. It passes through the placenta to the baby and should not be given within four hours of delivery. Excessive use of Scopolamine combined with narcotics is the reason why, in the past, in some American hospitals women in labour were put in high, barred, padded cots, wore helmets like those used by baseball players, or were tied in strait-jackets so that they could not damage themselves as a result of their restless and disturbed behaviour. Fortunately Scopolamine is now rarely used.

General anaesthesia

This sends the woman to sleep. It eradicates pain, but is the most hazardous method of pain relief for the mother and the baby because of the risk of inhaling vomit, the fourth most common cause of maternal death in the USA and Britain.[4] It is used for Caesarean birth, especially when done as an emergency, and occasionally for a difficult vaginal delivery or the birth of a second twin.

Ketamine is one fast-acting general anaesthetic, the effect of which lasts only five to ten minutes, which is also used intravenously in smaller doses for pain relief instead of narcotics. It can produce confusion, unpleasant dreams and hallucinations. It should never be used with sedatives or barbiturates. Though its safe use in obstetrics has not been established, it is claimed that its analgesic use – i.e., to reduce rather than eradicate pain – has no side-effects on the baby.[5]

Regional anaesthesia

This kills pain in one area of the body only. The great advantage of this method is that the mother is awake and aware and ready to greet her baby. There are many kinds of regional anaesthetics:

Paracervical block is used frequently in the USA, but rarely in Britain. It involves injecting into the cervix an anaesthetic similar to that used in dental surgery. Pain relief lasts for one to two hours and works well in seven out of ten women. The anaesthetic passes through the mother's bloodstream to the baby, causes temporary slowing of the fetal heart rate and may have subtle neurological effects on the baby in the period after birth.

Pudendal block entails anaesthetic being injected inside the vagina. It anaesthetizes the area around the vagina and between the vagina and anus, and may be used just before delivery. The effect lasts for about an hour. If it gets into the baby's bloodstream because delivery is not immediate it can cause respiratory depression.

With *spinal anaesthesia* anaesthetic is injected into the fluid around the spinal cord. Pain relief lasts for one to two hours. There is loss of sensation from the level of the breasts down. This means a greatly increased chance of forceps delivery since the woman does not get an urge to push the baby out and, because the pelvic floor muscles are slack from anaesthetic, the baby's head may not rotate into the correct position for birth. As a result it may get stuck. This is called deep transverse arrest.

8a The position of the needle when 8b The position of the needle for a
a paracervical block is given. pudendal nerve block.

Spinal anaesthesia can be used for Caesarean birth. The anaesthetic has
an indirect effect on the baby through changes in the mother's metabolism
and may also be present in the baby's bloodstream, resulting in subtle
neurological changes in the period after birth. A major problem with
spinal anaesthesia is that after the birth a woman may have a crashing
headache which can last as long as eight days, so that she cannot sit up,
or even shift position as she lies in bed. This occurs because of an escape of
cerebrospinal fluid. If the headache is severe a blood patch can be done by
injecting her own blood into the puncture hole, thus forming a clot which
closes it.

A *saddle-block* is a form of spinal anaesthesia in which the only part
anaesthetized is an area in the pelvis corresponding to the shape of a
saddle, which includes the lower abdomen, buttocks, perineum and inner
thighs. The effects and side-effects are similar to those of a spinal anaesthetic. It may be used for forceps deliveries and lasts for one and a half
to two hours. The saddle-block is commonly used in the USA but rarely in
Britain.

Extradural anaesthesia does not entail entering the fluid around the
spine; the injection stops short at the *dura*, a wall of tissue between the

8c   The position of the needle for a
saddle block (right).

8d   The position of the needle for a
caudal (below left).

8e   The position of the needle for a
continuous lumbar epidural (below
right).

vertebrae and the spinal canal. There are two main types, caudal and lumbar epidural:

Caudal anaesthesia entails an injection just below the sacrum, the bone in the small of the back. There is less paralysis than with a spinal and no risk of post-puncture headache. But the chance of forceps delivery is high for the same reasons as when a spinal is given. Any neurological effects in the baby are slight. A single dose lasts 45 minutes to an hour and a half.

An *epidural* is given at a higher point in the back. It requires less anaesthetic than a caudal and can be done so that it anaesthetizes only the area where pain is felt. Pain relief lasts for one to two hours. If done expertly a woman may retain feeling and some movement in her legs; however, many women lose all sensation.

With a *continuous lumbar epidural*, a fine plastic tube (a cannula) is inserted in the lower back between the vertebrae and into the epidural space around the spinal cord, and left in place. Top-ups can be given through this when needed.

A small test dose of the anaesthetic should always be given and the effects noted, before the full dose is introduced. If the anaesthetist seems to be spending a long time setting up the epidural, it is because great care must be taken. It may take half an hour to 45 minutes to give it.

The pros and cons of epidurals

For a woman who decides that she needs the help of drugs, an epidural is the most effective way of achieving complete relief from childbirth pain – and, indeed, possibly from all sensation, while remaining mentally alert. Even so, for two or three women out of every ten an epidural does not block all pain. It either does not work at all, or relieves rather than eradicates pain, or there are 'windows' in the area which the drug is intended to numb, often resulting in one-sided pain.[6]

Since an epidural service is available in most modern obstetric units, it may be worth discussing epidurals in more detail so that, depending on the circumstances and how you feel at the time, you can make a decision about what you want.

Some advantages of an epidural are:

- The baby is likely to be minimally affected by the drug. This is usually bupivacaine, a cocaine type of drug.[7]
- The woman's mind is unclouded to welcome her baby.

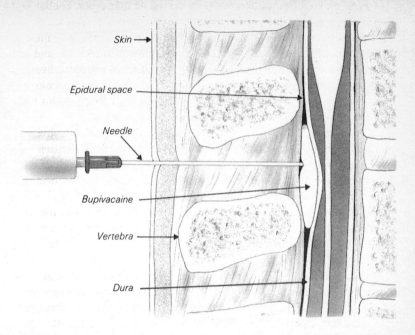

9 Tip of needle lying in epidural space. The dura is the membrane which forms the outer covering of the spinal cord. With an epidural, the needle must not penetrate the dura.

- When forceps or any other operative procedures are employed, no other method of anaesthesia has to be used.
- For Caesarean birth it is a method of anaesthesia in which the mother is able to be awake and to see her baby immediately. She does not have the unpleasant after-effects of general anaesthesia. If her blood pressure is very high an epidural reduces it to a safe level.
- When a woman is in pain and over-breathing, the relief from pain that comes from an epidural restores the balance between acid and alkaline elements in her blood, and also in that of her baby.[8]

Some disadvantages of an epidural are:

- The woman's blood pressure may drop excessively, making her feel faint, sick and giddy. Sometimes it plummets and other drugs must be given to raise it again, one reason why an intravenous catheter must be set up first. Having a drip in her arm is an inconvenience to the woman and limits her mobility.

- It tends to make the second stage of labour longer.[9] This is a problem where obstetricians impose set time-limits on the expulsive phase, and a woman may end up with a Caesarean section for this reason alone.

- Once an epidural is given, a woman may become a passive patient and receive further interventions which she had hoped to avoid. Because she cannot empty her bladder voluntarily a catheter is inserted to draw off urine. She must have an intravenous drip in her arm so that any negative effects of the drug can be immediately counteracted with other drugs. She receives continuous electronic fetal monitoring. If contractions slow down and get weaker, as they often do after an epidural has been given, a uterine stimulant may be used in the intravenous drip to force her uterus to contract more efficiently.

- The chances of forceps delivery are greatly increased.[10] This is partly because the woman may have no urge to push and so is unable to work with her body to get the baby born, and partly because the normal tone of the pelvic floor muscles through which the baby descends, its head rotating into the correct position for delivery as it does so, is destroyed by an epidural, so the baby may get stuck.

- Occasionally the needle punctures the dura (the membrane which encloses the spinal cord). This can result in escape of spinal fluid and a very severe headache after the birth – so bad that the woman has to lie flat and quite still for several days. If the drug solution is injected into the spine following accidental dural puncture, spinal rather than epidural anaesthesia is given. Since the dose for an epidural is much larger, this may lead to a sudden dramatic drop in blood pressure, difficulty in breathing (or, very occasionally, inability to breathe) and, very rarely, cardiac arrest.

- After the birth a woman who has had an epidural may have a greater blood loss than otherwise, and may have difficulty in emptying her bladder for some hours or days. Approximately three women in ten report this bladder problem. The urinary catheter may need to be left in place. She sometimes also experiences dizziness and 'ear-popping'.[11]

- There are some possible effects on the baby. Bupivacaine crosses the placenta into the baby's bloodstream within ten minutes and, after the baby is born, cord blood levels of the anaesthetic are 30 to 40 per cent of the mother's blood level.[12] It is often claimed that an epidural has no effect at all on the baby. It is true that it does not produce the problems with breathing and limpness that can result from pethidine, but it may have a more subtle effect on the baby's behaviour. The baby may be less responsive to the human voice, may have decreased motor maturity (muscle tone and strength) and be more irritable than babies of mothers who have no drugs. Various orienting and alerting skills tend to be depressed for as long as six weeks after birth.[13]

In spite of many articles in medical journals about epidurals, most studies are uncontrolled surveys. One obstetrician has summed up the state of current knowledge and its implications as follows:

> We have no way of knowing which of the reported results are really due to the epidural, and which are non-causally associated. In the absence of a randomized controlled trial, we are left with the uncomfortable realization that any differences reported might be due to differences in the women who choose to have or not to have an epidural, in the type of prenatal preparation they may have had, in the support they may have received in labor, or in other confounding variables which may influence the results, rather than to the procedure itself . . . However, even if strong evidence were available, it could only give us the statistical probabilities of various outcomes. Pain, suffering, enjoyment, control, sense of accomplishment, all have different meanings and values to each childbearing woman. She must weigh the available evidence according to her own value system, her own unique experience.[14]

A woman may very much want to give birth naturally but be unable to do so and be enormously grateful for the relief from pain an epidural can give. Maggie, for example, went to childbirth classes and was enthusiastic and confident about having a natural, unassisted birth. Unfortunately, she was 'overdue' and her doctor was worried about whether the baby was still growing. She was induced 14 days after term. She told me about her labour, with her baby in a posterior position:

> Contractions began two minutes apart, like they were testing me or trying to break my resolve. At the end of three hours I'd gone from two to three centimetres. I was vomiting, sweating and shaky. My legs would no longer let me walk. I was put on a syntocinon drip. I now admitted that I was at the

end of my tether. I had good rapport with the medical staff and felt I could trust them. They didn't mention an epidural. I said I wanted one.

I was given the anaesthetic quickly by a kindly anaesthetist who was sympathetic to my feelings. The fear and tension were soon gone. I felt waves of almost euphoric (and slightly sexual) passion with each contraction. After about four hours I suddenly began to PUSH. The anaesthetic was wearing off, I could feel pressure and contractions but no pain. The doctor and midwife were concerned that I should deliver normally and avoid episiotomy and forceps. Because of the anaesthetic I needed to be guided but it was no time before I could put my hand down and feel the baby's head just awaiting birth. I delivered my daughter with no assistance but lots of encouragement quietly and considerately given. I had a little skin tear which was sutured immediately while I held my baby and looked into her eyes.

In the months leading up to labour I prepared myself intensely and determinedly for a natural delivery and refused to even entertain the idea that anything might go wrong or be beyond me. I had to cross the barrier of anger and frustration before I could peaceably accept it. But my epidural made it possible for me to enjoy what would otherwise have been an exhausting, painful and distressing labour.

Handling pain with your own resources

Men, who are not going to actually physically give birth, but are onlookers and bystanders, have the feeling that they have got to *do* something about the pain, about the way labour is progressing, whereas women, who know that they will probably go through this experience, even if they have not already been through it, understand that it is a very important part of how a woman functions in life, and that there are worse things in life than pain, and that to go through the process of pregnancy and labour and be in control of it is a very important part of a woman's self-esteem (*Wendy Savage, the feminist obstetrician, in evidence to the tribunal investigating her management of five cases, February 1986*).

No pain-relieving drug is entirely free of risk. You may want to consider non-pharmaceutical ways of achieving pain relief. One anaesthetist claims that 30 per cent of women can benefit greatly from what he calls 'psychological analgesia', 10 per cent of them requiring no drugs at all and another 15 to 20 per cent needing fewer drugs because of their previous preparation.[15] And even those for whom pain is not diminished do not suffer in the same way because pain is not compounded by fear and anxiety.

For many women the pain of normal childbirth is qualitatively different from that of injury. It hurts, but that is a side-effect of a creative process, the powerfully working uterus. It is pain with a purpose. But even this pain can be shattering if you simply struggle to endure it.

Techniques for handling pain are not an end in themselves. They are a way of changing your level of consciousness – being in a state of what I call 'focused concentration' and what Michel Odent describes as 'being on another planet'.[16] It probably does not matter what you call it as long as you realize that it is not a question of 'doing exercises', or of 'distracting' yourself from pain, as is often suggested, but of going along with the experience and adapting yourself to the incredible power of your uterus.

Rhythmic, controlled breathing, relaxation and focused concentration are all ways of meeting pain and working with it, instead of trying to fight or escape from the sensations of labour. You will need to learn these in childbirth classes, as they are almost impossible to learn from a book. Whatever classes are available in your area, remember that good ones are not concerned only with pain prevention or the reduction of sensation. Other methods – hypnosis for example – may do this better. In a childbirth class you should find you become more self-assured, know how to work with your body and trust it, and are ready to start out on the exciting experience of birth with courage, confidence and energy. Classes teach you how to adjust yourself to your labour, whatever kind it may be, how to understand what your doctor or midwife are trying to do to help you, and provide a sort of map for childbirth, so that at any point you can take your bearings, tell approximately where you are, and see the part in its place in the whole. You will usually learn specific breathing and relaxing techniques, and how to adjust your posture and make special movements to help you handle contractions.

Many women who have been to classes would say that to have anaesthetics for normal childbirth is a bit like offering someone who is enjoying climbing a mountain, or a runner about to win a race, a whiff of something 'to ease the pain'. The aching muscles are all part of the hard work that the body is doing in a task in which you are totally involved, as you concentrate on 'riding over' each contraction carefully with breathing and neuro-muscular release. There is something enormously rewarding in the rhythms of labour, even above the joy of bringing new life into the world. When you really start to swim with the waves of contractions it can be a deeply satisfying experience. I remember feeling myself – and I am a far from athletic person – 'Oh, this is one sport I can really do!'

In classes you learn, with your future birth companion, how to relax while keeping your breathing rhythmic during powerful contractions. This is often done by 'lifting' breathing over the crest of each wave, allowing it to get quicker and lighter if you can no longer breathe slowly with comfort.

One way of doing this is to visualize a spiral staircase. When you are at the bottom of the staircase the breathing is slow and full, as if in big circles. When you need to, you go 'up' the spiral into smaller circles of quick, light breathing, ascending your spiral as far as you feel you need to go for that particular contraction, and then drop down again into slow, full breathing as it comes to an end.

Relaxation is sometimes taught as a drill, contracting the muscles of the left arm, right leg, right arm, left leg, both legs, and so on, and releasing them on command. That kind of teaching is unrelated to the actual patterns of muscle contraction in stress situations, and does little to help us become aware of how and why we tighten up. The new way is to teach relaxation as part of increased positive and pleasurable body awareness, closely linked with breathing.

One of my own approaches to relaxation is called Touch Relaxation. You learn to use touch as a signal for relaxation, and release in response to the warmth and pressure of your partner's hands. First you contract some of those muscles which are most likely to tighten at different stress phases of labour: your shoulders, back, neck and throat, abdominal muscles, inner thigh muscles, feet, buttock muscles, pelvic floor, and so on. As you deliberately hold the tension you note which other muscles have contracted at the same time. You also observe whether this tension has affected your breathing and, if so, how. At the same time, your partner notices how you look, so that he or she is aware of your appearance when tense. Your partner then rests hands firmly over the contracted muscles, and you release as if flowing out towards the hands. Your partner can feel the release of tension and so knows that the message given is effective. Even someone who lacks confidence about helping you realizes immediately that this works.

You will discover that certain kinds of touch are particularly effective. For many women firm foot-holding is useful, or your partner can use massage, stroking or holding to encourage relaxation. In labour he or she can sit holding your shoulders, breathing with you during difficult contractions and in continuous eye contact. The emotional support and encouragement that this gives is an advance on the kind of exercises in which a woman is supposed to fix her gaze on a spot on the wall while her partner stands by, timing contractions with a stop-watch.

Women were once prepared for the second stage of labour by being encouraged to tone and develop their abdominal muscles, and went into training in order to hold their breath for long periods. We now know that such gymnastics are not only irrelevant but can sometimes, as in the case of prolonged breath-holding, be dangerous. There is no advantage in being able to hold your breath for ten seconds or longer, and this practice may reduce the oxygen concentration in the blood available to the fetus, especially if you are also lying flat on your back, with resulting pressure on the inferior vena cava (big blood vessels in the lower part of your body).

A major change is also taking place in the way in which breathing and posture for the second stage is taught. My own teaching focuses on the idea of the 'unforced second stage', and aims to help women be aware of and respond to surges of desire to push which come like waves within each contraction, rather than training them to push for as long, as hard and as often as they can. The result is a less strenuous and more rhythmic, spontaneous way of handling contractions, without the need for cheerleaders urging the woman: 'Push! Come on! Don't waste your contraction! Push! Push!' Your partner can remind you to think of yourself opening up, keeping your mouth soft and relaxed and releasing muscles around your vagina. Each push is followed by shallow breathing until the next wave of desire to push builds up, when your breathing spontaneously becomes more staccato, culminating in the next automatically held breath as the baby moves down your vagina towards birth. This kind of breathing and relaxation, and the gentle approach to the second stage, is described in my books *The Experience of Childbirth, Pregnancy and Childbirth* and *Women's Experience of Sex* (see pp. 308–9 for details).

In many classes you can also learn the skills of visualization, so that you can link actively created, vivid pictures in your head with the feeling of opening up and letting go, a much more effective way of 'tuning in' to your body in childbirth than performing exercises.[17] I often describe the fanning open of the tissues of the perineum as like the petals of a peony unfolding, for example, with the baby's head like the hard bud in the centre. Focused concentration is another important element in handling pain with your own resources. Listening to your breathing is one way of doing this. Each breath in and out sounds like a wave washing on the shore, and focusing on the sound and image of the waves enables you to become more positively aware of your body. Some women find that it helps to make 'affirmations' – simple positive statements, or sometimes prayers – as they go through labour, not only to reduce sensations of pain but to have a positive effect on the body's energy and coordination through the power of the mind: 'I am strong . . . I accept the healthy pain that will birth my baby . . . My cervix is dilating more and more.' An Orthodox Jewish woman I know said over and over again, 'Gates of Jerusalem, open for me!' (And they did!)

A woman who has her sexual partner sharing the birth experience with her may find not only that the very fact of her lover's presence and emotional support gives her strength, but that being held, stroked and embraced releases tension and enables pain to become a sensation she can 'go with', and even enjoy.

There are good physiological reasons for this. Though it may seem that making love is the last thing a woman would want to do if she were in pain, you may have noticed that erotic arousal can temporarily obliterate the pain of toothache or a headache, for example. Many women have found that love-making can ease both premenstrual tension and menstrual pain. This is not only because it helps relaxation, but because they feel suffused with the peace and satisfaction – difficult to describe – which somehow softens pain so that, though it may still be there in the background, it seems unimportant. This is because sexual arousal stimulates the release of natural pain-killers in the body which are chemically related to opium.[18] As you become more and more sexually excited, these endorphins pour into your bloodstream to change what may seem like sheer, overwhelming hard work or an endurance test into a thrilling experience in which pain is there, but can no longer dominate you.

Sexual arousal in childbirth also releases oestrogen into your circulation. This helps the uterus to contract effectively, speeds up labour and, if uterine action has been uncoordinated, can get your uterus working better and enable the cervix to open more easily. When there is more effective uterine function, with the upper part of the uterus strong and the lower part soft and opening, pain is reduced, even though contractions get stronger.

Many women would not want to make love during labour but the whole of childbirth is for them a psycho-sexual experience. The energy produced by the uterus, the feeling of the baby's head pressing down and all the tissues fanning out and opening up – these sensations are in themselves felt as sexual, and produce the same joyous feelings that might come from being held and caressed by a lover. Endorphins and oestrogen flood through the woman's body to coordinate the action of the uterus and to change her perception of pain.[19]

Many other techniques have now been introduced into childbirth education which, either directly or indirectly contribute towards the relief of pain. Acupressure – shiatsu – can also be very helpful, for example, not so much as a system by itself, but incorporated with other ways of giving comfort and finding harmony with what is happening in your body. There are specific points on the feet, buttocks and wrist, for instance, where firm pressure can help a woman cope with labour pains, and this can be linked with massage. Teachers who have attended my own workshops in body awareness in childbirth often use these techniques with their childbirth classes. Others have studied Chinese shiatsu, and sometimes acupuncture too, and have a systematic approach based on oriental philosophies of healing.

Most acupuncturists who work with women in childbirth say that it is wrong to see acupuncture simply as a means of pain relief. They usually ask you to start treatment during pregnancy because they are concerned to help your body work harmoniously and to establish the right physical conditions for a positive experience of labour.

Ice massage is similar to acupuncture. It not only produces local constriction of blood vessels and makes the area numb, but can relieve pain for a long time after these effects have disappeared.[20] In labour it is sometimes useful over the lower back.

Transcutaneous electronic nerve stimulation (TENS) is another kind of analgesia which results from intense stimulation of the skin. Two pairs of electrodes are connected to a small battery-operated stimulator and the woman controls the electrical impulse herself, producing sharp bursts of pulsed buzzing as pain increases. The electrodes are supposed to be taped into position at either side of the spine. In fact, it is worth experimenting with them at different sites; sometimes having a pair on the thighs, feet or at other points of the body is still more helpful. In two Swedish hospitals where TENS was tested in childbirth 44 per cent of women said they had good or very good relief from pain using this method, another 44 per cent had some relief and 12 per cent said it did not help them.[21]

Hypnosis, whether it is the kind you use yourself or powerful suggestion introduced by someone else, can also be helpful for some women in childbirth. Though it can work satisfactorily without being practised beforehand, it is best to start hypnosis about half-way through pregnancy, because you then discover well in advance whether you are a good hypnotic subject and can become confident that it is an effective technique.

238 · The Way Birth Is

It provides complete relief from pain for approximately 20 per cent of women. And many others discover that it takes the edge off pain and reduces the quantity of pain-relieving drugs they require.[22]

Yoga, which offers the breathing awareness that comes with practising it regularly, and knowledge of positions in which the pelvis is wide, can also increase trust in your body and bring the strength that comes from self-confidence. You may be able to find classes of yoga for pregnancy, with a teacher who has special knowledge of childbirth, since the positions, movements and types of breathing used during labour need to be related to the specific stresses you are feeling then. This entails the teacher having a good understanding of the physiology of childbirth, and of how it feels to be in labour.[23]

There are many other non-pharmacological ways of relieving pain, giving comfort and increasing psycho-physical coordination in childbirth: the use of heat (hot compresses, a hot water bottle tucked in the small of your back, between your legs or over your lower abdomen, warm water – either floating in it or having it flowing over you[25]); distraction techniques (such as slowly counting backwards from ten); or what appears to be the opposite of this, the removal of all external distractions and being in a quiet, darkened room where you can surrender yourself completely to the enveloping experience without any interruptions;[24] or rhythmic sound, in the form of music, singing or chanting – it is said that one of the queens of France gave birth singing the Magnificat!

You will probably think that some of these methods could not possibly be right for you, but there is good evidence that every one of them works for some women. Pain is diminished, energy is released and everything the woman is feeling in labour is coordinated into a total experience which has pattern and meaning for her. There is a range of alternatives to using drugs for pain relief and it is wise to select several which you think would suit you, so that if one approach is insufficient other methods can be used to reinforce it. This sense of flexibility and the opportunity for choice can be empowering and may itself contribute to reduced perception of pain.

At this stage it may be a good idea to look back over all the methods of handling pain described in this chapter and note down some thoughts about each. Do you need to find out more about any of them? If so, how will you do this?

Then write about your own preferences, thinking both in terms of a labour that is going well, and also how you would want to handle pain if the going proved difficult.

Which methods, from your present vantage point, would you decide against? Make a note of these and the questions you want to raise with your doctor or midwife about each of them. Discuss this with your birth companion too, as it is important that this person understands exactly what you want.

For a woman expecting her first baby, the question of how she is going to manage pain tends to loom large in her thoughts. But the second time round she is often more concerned to negotiate beforehand to avoid all the irritating interference which is itself a cause of pain, so that she can give birth in her own way, in her own time and in peace.

OBSTETRICALLY DIRECTED BIRTH

The idea behind obstetric direction of labour is to improve on nature and get control over what can sometimes be an unpredictable, painful, long-drawn-out and occasionally even disastrous process. One obstetrician who takes this view writes:

> The natural childbirth groups fail to understand that the practice of medicine consists of the recognition and correction of the shortcomings of nature – nature is a bad midwife. Childbirth has become safer because of increasingly sophisticated methods of diagnosis and treatment. With the illogicality of women these are the very procedures they wish to discard . . . They insist that birth is a natural phenomenon but, equally, so is death.[1]

Kieran O'Driscoll, in Dublin, believes that complete obstetric control in labour, as distinct from a 'wait and see' attitude, reduces the amount of intervention needed later, makes the mother more comfortable and, in his hospital, cuts down the number of forceps and Caesarean deliveries to an impressively low 10 per cent and 4 per cent. He aims at a labour lasting not more than eight hours and promises each woman that she will not be in labour for more than twelve hours. If the rate of dilatation of the cervix falls below the norm, labour is speeded up with an oxytocin drip. Oxytocin is usually called pitocin in the USA, Syntocinon in Britain; these are artificial forms of the hormone which makes the uterus contract. Four out of every ten women having their first baby receive uterine stimulation of this kind.[2]

The Dublin approach is probably obstetrically directed labour at its best, with one-to-one nursing care and careful explanation to the woman of everything that is happening. But a good deal of obstetric management is at a much inferior level, and in O'Driscoll's words: 'Labour is made even more arduous for mothers by the introduction of invasive procedures practised in the name of the child, often with scant evidence as to their real value.'[3] Failed inductions – which end up in Caesarean sections – are a case in point. The routine use of pethidine and epidural anaesthesia is another, for 'benefits . . . are reaped almost entirely during the first stage of labour and the price paid largely during the second stage'.[4] That price is an increased chance of forceps delivery or Caesarean section. All these things turn a normal physiological process into an obstetric emergency.

So there is high-quality obstetrically directed labour, with each woman having her own personal midwife and continuity of care, on the one hand, and on the other a type of autocratic and invasive obstetric management which provides fragmented care and routinely interferes with the natural process of labour and introduces unnecessary risks.

Induction

Doctors have been intervening in childbirth ever since theories about labour based on the laws of mechanics were developed and methods of manipulating the fetus and enlarging the birth canal were devised in the hospital-schools of Paris in the early sixteenth century. But they were often spectacularly unsuccessful. They have been able to chemically control labour only in the last 20 years, with the invention of synthetic oxytocin. And it is only in the last five years or so that pessaries of prostaglandin, another hormone, have been used to soften and ripen the cervix and start labour.

Some obstetricians have definite rules as to which women should have labour induced: those with breech babies or who are diabetic at 36 or 38 weeks, for example; anyone who is two weeks over her expected date, or, depending on the obstetrician, ten days – or one week. Some insist that all women over 35 should be induced on the expected date, or even earlier. A slight rise in diastolic blood pressure to 90 may also be an indication for induction. You can ask about your doctor's policy on induction. A rate of more than 10 per cent is high.

Induced labours have disadvantages. They tend to be more painful, so induction starts a process in which powerful pain-killing drugs may have to be given. These in turn slow down labour and may lead to a forceps delivery. Induced labours are more likely than spontaneous labours to end in a Caesarean section.

When oxytocin is used, the fetal heart should be continuously monitored in case strong contractions are making labour too difficult for the baby and insufficient oxygenated blood is flowing through the umbilical cord and placenta into its bloodstream. The combination of an intravenous drip and continuous electronic fetal monitoring prevents a woman from moving around freely.

After an induced labour the baby may be discovered to be immature. Though a scan at 16 weeks helps to date pregnancy, babies are still sometimes hurled into the world before they are ready. Doctors often warn a woman that she must be induced because otherwise the baby will be too big to pass easily through her pelvis, but then find that it is of average, or even below average, weight.

The introduction of prostaglandin pessaries means that now more women can have their labours induced and still have a chance of vaginal delivery, because prostaglandin softens the cervix and makes it ready to open up. Even so, prostaglandins fail to induce labour in two out of every three women if the cervix is not naturally 'ripe'.

You do not have to agree to induction unless you are convinced that there is a strong reason to go into labour as soon as possible. Social reasons for induction – that your doctor is going away on holiday or your mother is coming to stay, for example – are no justification for interfering with the birth process.

Induction can help, however, if a woman has severe pre-eclampsia or any other condition in which it could be dangerous for the baby to be left inside longer, because it is not being nourished well in the uterus. One sign of this – which you can observe yourself if you stand on the scales at the same time each week – would be that you are actually losing, rather than gaining, weight. Otherwise the safest course of action is to wait patiently, keep a record of fetal movements and look forward to the spontaneous onset of labour.[5]

In up to 12 per cent of pregnancies the bag of waters bursts at some time during the hours or days preceding the start of active labour, and amniotic fluid leaks out.[6] As we have seen already, induction for premature rupture of the membranes is usually unnecessary. The chances of infection can be much reduced by not having vaginal examinations until labour is well under way, and even then having as few as possible.

> Make a note of anything else you want to find out about induction and acceleration of labour – e.g., other women's experiences of it, and the standard practice of hospitals in the area. Your childbirth teacher would be a good resource person and you may want to do some further reading.[7]

Clock-watched labour

Obstetric management goes along with high-technology childbirth. But there is one item of technology which, often overlooked because it is ancient, forms the basis of all the intervention which takes place – the clock.

The progress of dilatation per hour, the number of minutes between contractions and the length of each, the time from 2 cms to full dilatation (10 cm), and then from full dilatation to delivery, the time the head is on the perineum, the time of active pushing, and the timing of the third stage – from delivery of the baby till delivery of the placenta – are all watched and scrutinized, often with anxiety, and recorded on the labour chart.

Yet, obstetric management aside, time is often also important to the woman in labour. Women often ask: 'How long will it be?' 'When will the baby be born?' 'How long will contractions like this last?' 'When do you think I will go into the second stage?' 'How many more hours of this?' They are all questions which care-givers cannot answer honestly with any precision unless they manage labour with aggressive intervention. It means that they often feel under great pressure from the woman to help get the labour over.

But it is not such a simple matter as women wanting labour to be fast. Some women cope well with a tumultuous labour lasting only a few hours but are shattered by a long one. Others are shocked by a short, sharp labour which they feel has 'run away' with them, but can handle well a longer, more slowly unfolding labour – especially if they have some method of alleviating the backache which is often experienced in this kind of labour.

With any labour which takes more than about six hours, women are often made anxious by those caring for them about the time it is lasting. This anxiety makes labour more difficult and, by triggering the production of large amounts of the stress hormones epinephrine and norepinephrine, can interfere with its progress. There is a kind of time-lessness about a labour that is going well, whether short or long. The woman is immersed in the reality of her own experience, and nothing else matters.

Fetal monitoring

The baby's heart rate can be monitored intermittently by hand with a fetoscope (a special stethoscope) or trumpet, or using ultrasound or electronically to get a continuous tracing. With electronic fetal monitoring (EFM) signals are picked up and fed into a computer that measures and records them, producing results on a long print-out.

On the print-out – the CTG (cardiotocographic) tracing – the upper line records the baby's heart-beat, while the lower line shows the baby's movements. The normal heart rate is between 120 and 160 beats per

10   Woman connected to electronic fetal monitor.

minute, but the time between heart-beats varies (the 'beat-to-beat variation'), so the line zig-zags. Normally there is a variation of 5 to 10 beats per minute, but if the baby is asleep or drowsy from pethidine or other narcotic drugs received from your bloodstream, it may be less. When the baby kicks, or when you have a vaginal examination or shift position, the heart rate may speed up.

In some labours it is sensible to have continuous monitoring – for example if:
- you have an oxytocin intravenous infusion producing very powerful and frequent contractions;
- labour starts more than three weeks before the baby is due;
- there are signs that the baby has not grown well in the uterus and is likely to be frail;
- you have had any serious problem during pregnancy (e.g., diabetes, severe pre-eclampsia, a very high temperature);
- there is meconium in the amniotic fluid;
- abnormalities are discovered on listening to the baby's heart rate intermittently.

One advantage of EFM is that it gives you the reassurance that all is well with the baby – *if* the machine is working properly and *if* your baby conforms to a norm. But machines cannot always be relied on and babies sometimes look as if they are in trouble but turn out to be in good condition at birth. Another advantage of EFM is that it allows you and your birth companion to know when contractions are coming and be ready to adapt to each one.

There are two main types of machine. With the external monitor you have two tight bands round your abdomen to which are attached a couple of discs, one recording the heart-beat and the other the pressure of contractions. The second type is internal and consists of a small wire screw like a miniature corkscrew, or a clip like a staple, which is fixed to the baby's scalp, together with a pressure balloon – a tube filled with

11 Fetal scalp electrodes.

liquid – inside your uterus to record the length and strength of contractions.

The first method of monitoring may be safer because it is less invasive. It can be used when the membranes are still intact. But it is also less accurate. And it is impossible to move about when you are strapped up like this. Even shifting to get more comfortable on the bed interferes with the print-out, so you may be told to lie quite still. This causes aches and pains – and probably would even if you were not having a baby.

Sometimes the print-out is only clear when a woman is lying on her back. But this position is dangerous in labour because the uterus may press on large blood vessels in the lower part of your body and slow down the return of blood to your heart. This will make you feel sick, dizzy and faint and reduce the blood flowing through to the baby. In this way EFM can cause the very conditions it is designed to reveal.

The second method, with the scalp clip, may also immobilize you, though it is easier to move because you do not have tight bands round your abdomen, and since the electrode is fixed to the baby's head, it cannot shift away from it. But the monitor cannot be put in place until the membranes have ruptured, and this is sometimes given as a reason for artificially rupturing them. Amniotomy enables a clip to be put on the baby's scalp, and allows the doctor to see whether or not the fluid is clear. (The presence of meconium, the baby's first bowel movements, in amniotic fluid may be a sign that the baby is under excessive stress.)

On the other hand, once the membranes have ruptured the protective cushioning of fluid in front of the baby's head, around the cord through which the blood flows to the baby, and over the fetal surface of the placenta, is reduced. In most labours in which there is no intervention the membranes do not rupture spontaneously till towards the end of the first stage, usually not until the cervix has dilated by about 9 cm. When they are ruptured early, the baby's head is exposed to the effects of uneven pressure during contractions and the parietal bones – the skull bones, which are like a cap divided in the middle by a suture and a fontanelle (soft spot) at the front – may become misaligned and a swelling, called a *caput*, can develop under the scalp.[8] This is usually harmless, but is occasionally a sign that there has been bruising deeper down – and the brain lies directly beneath.

There is a third kind of continuous monitoring – *telemetry*. With this method, radio waves record the fetal heart rate and you do not need to be immobilized. The machinery can be put in your pocket as you walk about, and the recording picked up in another room some distance away. Telemetry is not in general use, however, and when it is available the woman is still often kept in bed. This is not necessary: a similar system is in fact used by zoologists to monitor the heart rates of wild birds and animals.

There is no evidence that routine monitoring saves babies' lives.[9] And it can certainly make birth more difficult for the mother, because there is a greater chance of Caesarean section, which brings its own risks.[10] Whether or not a woman has a Caesarean section, she is also more likely to acquire an infection and this risk increases the longer monitoring continues.[11] Many babies delivered by forceps or Caesarean section because EFM indicated fetal distress are actually in vigorous condition at birth and need not have had operative delivery.[12] Signs of apparent distress may have been picked up because their heads were squeezed or because they were drowsy from pain-killing drugs received through the mother's bloodstream.[13]

Electronic monitoring is sometimes used together with scalp blood analysis. If there seem to be heart rate abnormalities the baby's head is pricked and some blood drawn off and analysed. This offers a guide as to whether or not that baby ought to be delivered immediately by forceps or Caesarean section. When these two methods of assessing fetal well-being are used together, convulsions can be prevented in several babies in every thousand.[14] It is not known whether convulsions have any long-term effects on babies, though it would seem better to avoid them if possible. But there is a price to pay. That price is being strapped up or having a wire stuck in the baby's head (with the slight risk of a scalp abscess), being more or less immobilized, having many other kinds of intervention when the monitor does not work properly or the print-out is wrongly interpreted, and an increased risk of forceps delivery or Caesarean section.

> Record your thoughts about electronic fetal monitoring and anything you wish to find out more about from your doctor or midwife.

Amniotomy

Many obstetricians and midwives practise routine artificial rupture of the membranes as soon as the woman is admitted to hospital and seems to be in labour, or at 3 or 4 cm dilatation of the cervix, whether or not they wish to put an electrode on the baby's head.

Advantages are that if the baby has passed meconium into the amniotic fluid, showing that it *may* be in trouble, this can be seen; it also allows access to the baby's scalp for blood analysis and electronic monitoring of the fetal heart rate, and may make labour shorter if the cervix is already ripe.

But there are disadvantages. In many hospitals it is the rule that once the waters have broken delivery must take place within 12 hours (or 24, depending on your obstetrician). If you don't deliver by then it will be a Caesarean birth, and if it looks as if you are not going to deliver within these time-limits, labour may be artificially speeded up. Amniotic fluid lubricates the baby, the cord and the membranes. So it protects the baby's head, prevents the cord being squashed and helps blood flow freely between the placenta and the baby. There may be a lot of pressure against the cord, the placenta and the baby's head during strong contractions after the membranes have ruptured, and the heart rate may slow down. If membranes are ruptured when the presenting part is high, the cord, or an arm, may drop down.[15]

You may decide that amniotomy should not be done unless your doctor or midwife can convince you that it will be helpful in your particular labour, either because there is reason to be concerned about the condition of the baby and they want to insert a scalp electrode, or because labour is taking a very long time, you are already half dilated, and amniotomy may trigger the extra spurt of uterine activity you need.

The intravenous drip

Having an intravenous drip set up so that drugs and fluids can be introduced straight into your bloodstream is another procedure that forms part of the obstetric management of labour. Some obstetricians believe that a vein should always be opened and fluids dripped in so that the woman does not get dehydrated and drugs can be introduced straight into her bloodstream in an emergency. They consider it better for her to receive intravenous glucose than to be allowed to eat or drink, in case she has to have general anaesthesia for Caesarean section, when she might inhale her stomach contents.

But in ensuring against one risk, this kind of obstetric management exposes you and the baby to two others. The first is water intoxication, when an excess of fluids in the body upsets its chemical balance. If severe, this could lead to brain damage. Water intoxication is more likely to occur if you are also having pethidine, oxytocin or continuous epidural anaesthesia, since they decrease the flow of urine. The other risk involves the intravenous fluid used, which is usually dextrose, a glucose solution. In the USA high concentrations are given – 20 to 30 per cent – while in Britain a much lower concentration of 10 per cent is the norm. There may be problems for the baby with high concentrations of sugar, because dextrose crosses the placenta and if the baby is born with a high level of sugar in the bloodstream, but this is not kept up after birth, it can become hypoglycaemic – that is, the blood sugar can drop to an abnormal level. This is one cause of convulsions. (A British anaesthetist, Professor Selwyn Crawford, has stated that intravenous sugar solution is a 'poison'.[16])

Even if a dextrose intravenous drip is not used routinely on every woman, it is common practice to order one if a woman's blood sugar drops in labour. During pregnancy you store more sugar than usual in your bloodstream to meet your baby's needs. If you don't have food in labour, but are using a lot of energy – especially if labour is long – you get short of sugar and start to burn fat. If you don't drink you are also likely to get dehydrated. Starvation plus dehydration produces ketosis. Acids called 'ketones' build up in your bloodstream and you have a headache, get drowsy and tend to overbreathe. Ketosis is much more common than needing general anaesthesia for emergency Caesarean section, so it would seem that avoiding starvation and dehydration by eating and drinking when you wish is a sensible course to follow.

If you develop ketosis you could have either an intravenous dextrose drip or glucose drinks. In one hospital which has stopped setting up intravenous drips for ketosis, it has been discovered that ketones disappear from urine after a while if a woman has plenty of sweet drinks. So it is important to eat and drink when you want. Most women do not want to eat once labour is well established, and if they do, or if their stomach is already overloaded, they vomit. On the other hand, in the early phases before your cervix is half-dilated, you may enjoy low-residue foods which are easily digested: soup, smooth vegetable and fruit purées and honey (not milk or high-fibre vegetables). Your natural thirst is a good guide to when and how much to drink. Iced water, sweetened juices or lemon tea can be very pleasant. In strong labour the gut shuts down, but you can still absorb glucose in liquid. Most women also enjoy sucking ice cubes.

This is another subject to discuss with your doctor or midwife. Make a note of questions you want to ask both concerning their general practice and what they do if ketones appear in the urine.

Episiotomy

When the crown of the baby's head pushes against the tissues of the perineum and can be seen like a wrinkled walnut just inside the vagina, surgical intervention is usually made – episiotomy. This is an incision in the perineum to enlarge the vaginal outlet. It was introduced by obstetricians when they took over from midwives, and has now become one of the routine procedures of childbirth, performed on the majority of women having first babies – and many having second and subsequent babies too. When DeLee in the twenties first recommended the practice of routine episiotomy and forceps delivery he claimed that this would prevent the fetal head becoming a 'battering ram' and suffering prolonged pounding and congestion leading to brain damage.[17]

No proof for this kind of statement has ever been produced. In a randomized control trial at the Rotunda Hospital in Dublin babies were in an

Mid-line episiotomy

12 Medio-lateral episiotomy. The dotted line shows where a mid-line episiotomy is made. In Britain medio-lateral episiotomies are usually done, in the USA mid-line episiotomies.

equally good condition at birth whether their mothers had episiotomy, a tear or an intact perineum.[18]

There is also the woman to consider. Women's feelings about episiotomy have hardly been investigated at all. Instead there are numerous studies on different ways of performing episiotomy and methods of suturing afterwards. In the few research projects in which women have been asked what they think, enquiry has usually been restricted to how they feel during the six weeks after childbirth, and often only in the first week. Most doctors do not realize that women can have problems with episiotomy and suturing of the perineum for months, and sometimes even years, after.

My own research [19] indicated that women are often shocked by the pain they experience. Many have stitches which are supposed to dissolve but do not and which eventually either have to be removed or become embedded in scar tissue. Some are sutured so tightly that there is no space for the swelling of tissue which always follows injury. They often say they cannot sit easily when holding the baby and it is especially difficult when breastfeeding. Some women are left with painful lumps of scar tissue months after birth and sexual intercourse is extremely painful – or impossible. Only 22 per cent of the episiotomy mothers said that intercourse was comfortable within the first month compared with 39 per cent of those with tears and 64 per cent of those who had no injury to the perineum. Women with episiotomies tended to have pain which lasted longer than three months.

Further studies have since been done which also demonstrate that episiotomy is often performed unnecessarily, causes pain both at delivery and in the weeks after, and makes intercourse uncomfortable.[20] Episiotomy might be worth it if it had long-term benefits, but there is no evidence that it does anything to improve the condition of a woman's perineum or her pelvic muscles, and it certainly sometimes causes sexual problems.

Though there are situations in which a baby has to be born quickly, and then episiotomy is done for a practical reason, from an anthropological point of view most episiotomies serve a ritual function, and mark with a dramatic flourish the significance of the act of delivery by genital mutilation of the mother.

There is now growing awareness among obstetricians and midwives that far too many episiotomies are done, and women having babies are asking searching questions about this surgical intervention.[21]

If you decide you want to avoid episiotomy, discuss the subject with your doctor or midwife well before labour starts. You can say that you do not want an episiotomy unless you are forewarned, are given an explanation of why you need one and have agreed to it. You may want this written in your notes. Practise pelvic floor exercises, especially the lift exercise (pp. 59–60). Concentrate on feeling your perineum bulge down like a heavy bag of soft fruit. Also practise light, rather quick breathing with your mouth open while you feel soft and loose below. This helps during contractions as the baby is sliding out. Regularly massage the skin in and around your vagina with warm oil and concentrate on visualizing yourself open while you do this. Ask whoever is supporting you in labour to use the word 'open' rather than 'push'. Push only when you most want to, and only as hard as you want to. Remind the person attending you that you would like to deliver without an episiotomy. When you feel the baby's head pressing through your vagina and beginning to stretch you wide open, rest your fingers lightly on the head and get into a position where you can look down and see the birth of your baby. That way you will realize when it is sensible to stop pushing and start *breathing* the baby out instead.

Caesarean section

By Caesarean section the obstetrician achieves ultimate control over birth. He cuts another, artificial orifice and lifts the baby out. Through the act of surgery he has acquired the female power of giving birth. It is his expertise, his surgical skill which produces the baby.

In the seventies the American Caesarean rate increased threefold and now almost one woman in five has a Caesarean birth. Though rates are lower in Europe, there is virtually an epidemic of Caesarean sections throughout the Western world. Analysis of the US increase gives a good indication of the reasons why most Caesareans are done.[22]

The most frequent reason is that *labour is slow* –'dystocia'. Thirty per cent of the rise in Caesarean section has been attributed to dystocia. So if you would prefer to avoid Caesarean section think ahead about how you would cope with a long, tiring labour: freedom to walk about and get in the shower or bath to relax, being given a lot of encouragement, and above all, *not being hurried*.

Repeat Caesareans comprise another 25 to 30 per cent of the increase. A repeat Caesarean section is often done because there is concern that the scar from the previous operation may rupture, so if you want to have a vaginal birth after a previous Caesarean section (VBAC), say that you do not wish your labour to be augmented with oxytocin, as this increases the risk of that happening.

Breech births are responsible for 10 to 15 per cent of the increase. When a baby is born bottom-first there is a chance of hold-up with the delivery of the head – the widest part of the body – and resulting lack of oxygen. Caesarean section for a breech birth should not be necessary if:

- You have a normal pelvis.
- The baby is expected to weigh less than 8 lbs.
- The baby is curled up into a ball with its head forward on to its chest – *a frank breech.*

Fetal distress accounts for another 10 to 15 per cent of the increase. This diagnosis is made more often when electronic monitoring is used. As a result Caesarean section rates tend to go up threefold when monitoring starts being used in the hospital, but fall later when there is experience with interpretation of the print-out. There are steps you can take to ensure that your baby gets enough oxygen: be well nourished, in good health and rested when labour starts; decline induction and oxytocin stimulation; avoid drugs in labour; move about, and when you want to lie down, do so on your side rather than your back; breathe rhythmically, stay relaxed, rest between contractions; have emotional support so that you stay confident and calm; in the second stage choose upright positions and avoid prolonged breath-holding and frantic straining.

The disadvantages of Caesarean section are that it:

- Increases the risk of birth for the mother (the mortality rate is almost four times as high as for vaginal birth), largely from the effects of general anaesthesia.
- Is more likely than a vaginal birth to result in infection (sometimes a risk as high as 65 per cent). Infection may occur in the lining of the uterus, the urinary tract and the wound itself.
- When mistimed, leads to the birth of a pre-term baby, with all the associated risks of prematurity.
- Is more likely to result in the delivery of a baby who has breathing difficulties after birth, whether or not the baby is premature. This may be because uterine contractions and the passage through the birth canal squeeze out excess fluid from the lungs and massage the baby to provide an important respiratory stimulus.

- Introduces additional risk of rupture (separation in the muscle wall) of the uterus in future births. With a lower-segment transverse incision rather than a vertical incision, however, this risk is slight.

Though we may think of Caesarean sections as being done to save babies' lives, they are often performed for less pressing reasons, and a great many may not be necessary.

If a Caesarean section is on the cards but you hope to deliver vaginally, you will need to bring this into the open with your doctor, discuss it fully and have a birth plan which reflects the outcome of this discussion. You will be asking for a 'trial of labour'. This takes place when it is not known whether or not a woman can deliver vaginally, and is conducted in hospital with everything ready for a Caesarean section if necessary. It is a trial of the uterus and not of the woman having the baby! Obstetricians are increasingly reluctant to allow a trial of labour and advise, or insist on, an elective (planned in advance) Caesarean section because they believe it is safer.

This is happening particularly often when there is a breech presentation. Sometimes a woman is told that if she insists on trying for vaginal birth she will end up with a brain-damaged baby. This is just a threat and is not supported by the facts. A Canadian follow-up study of breech babies which followed the children until they were 8 years old concluded: 'There appears to be no difference in the subsequent health and development of breech infants whether delivered vaginally or by Caesarean section.'[23]

Bear in mind, however, that if you have an oddly shaped or very small pelvis, or if the breech baby is likely to be very big, or has its legs extended, a Caesarean birth may be safer in the end. Suppose that after detailed discussion you decide that Caesarean section would be wiser – what then? You need not simply hand over to your obstetrician. Discuss the different ways in which the operation could be done and different kinds of anaesthesia. Let your doctor know the things that are most important to you about the birth and the time afterwards. One vital aspect of good care in birth, as we have seen already, is being able to have someone with you who is on the same wavelength and gives strong and loving emotional support. That holds good whether or not you have a vaginal birth, and in many ways a woman who is having Caesarean section needs that support even more urgently than when labour is proceeding normally. Contact one of the Caesarean birth organizations listed on p. 311 for further information, and work out a birth plan which meets your needs (see pp. 292–3).

CEREMONIAL BIRTH PROCEDURES

Ever since the mid-eighteenth century, when maternity hospitals were first established in England for the indigent poor so that doctors could practise on them, ceremonial procedures have accumulated which regulate everything that happens inside a hospital. These rules often erect a rigid barrier between the woman in childbirth and those attending her, and make her the passive object of care.

In those first charity hospitals the patients were poor, powerless – and female. The doctors were powerful, comfortably off – and male. As professional men they were separated by the gulf of social class not only from their impoverished patients but also from the nurses, who came from the working class, and they treated them accordingly. Midwives were not employed in these hospitals, since it was probable that they would have known a great deal more about childbirth than the doctors. Instead nurses were engaged who would be sure to defer to doctors and take orders from them.

Specialist doctors, the majority of them male, are still at the top of the hospital hierarchy, controlling both the patients at the bottom and the female nurses who carry out their orders. Rules and regulations provide what is intended to be a standard setting for birth, often prevent the exercise of individual initiative by any member of staff, and attempt to ensure that every patient is treated in exactly the same way.

Most routine procedures performed on women in childbirth are of only marginal benefit to them. Some make labour more uncomfortable and difficult. But they are part of the immutable ceremonial order of the hospital. And if these ceremonies are ignored or neglected, many members of staff are anxious that chaos and confusion will result. Sometimes these ritual procedures, even when of no practical help, make patients feel secure too.

In addition to their social function of regulating behaviour in the hospital, these ceremonies are also part of the armour with which some doctors, nurses and midwives protect themselves from the anxiety experienced when dealing with the dangerous passages and major life crises of birth, sickness and death. The initiation every medical student goes through – learning to dissect a corpse and not see it as a dead person, but as a collection of anatomical parts – is part of a training process which tends to screen out the doctor's awareness of the patient as an individual. In much the same way, as a houseman the doctor learns to perform ceremonies in obstetrics that depersonalize the woman and because they make initiative and decision-making unnecessary, reduce the anxiety provoked by uncertainty.[1]

Task-oriented rather than woman-oriented care encourages caregivers both to deny their own feelings and to detach themselves from any personal contact with patients which might prove threatening.[2] Perhaps this is why even when research shows that a procedure is unnecessary, causes discomfort or distress to the mother or can actually be dangerous, it continues to be performed. This chapter looks at some of these unnecessary ceremonies and customs.

Admission to hospital and the environment

Shaving

On admission to hospital it has been general practice to prepare the patient by shaving her perineal hair. This was first done in the nineteenth century to poor women who were having their babies in charity hospitals, to get rid of lice. It preceded the introduction of antiseptic procedures by Lister.

Studies showing that it was useless were first done in the 1960s.[3] Doctors were very nervous about undertaking any research on this subject. In one Californian study, women who were not going to be shaved were made to wash between their legs with pHisoHex for a whole month before delivery.[4]

It was not until the eighties that a midwife researcher, Mona Romney, showed that not only did shaving have no effect on infection, but it produced great discomfort for women after the birth, with itching and burning as the hair started to grow again. She concluded: 'Most patients disliked shaving and we can present no evidence to support its continued use . . . We believe that perineal shaving is an unjustified assault and should be abandoned.'[5]

Subsequent investigations with scanning electron microscopes reveal that shaving, even by skilled hands, always produces nicks in the skin which may be invisible to the naked eye and can be entry points for micro-organisms and are therefore a focus for infection, even if there is no episiotomy or tearing. An editorial in the *Lancet* advises: 'Since pre-operative shaving increases the rate of post-operative wound infection, this traditional surgical practice should be dropped.'[6]

The enema

Another routine admission procedure is the giving of an enema (or suppositories) to empty the lower bowel. The idea behind this is to avoid contamination of the perineum by faeces. Most women dislike it intensely and some have said that the pain produced by a large, strong enema was worse than any pain they had from contractions. Research shows that 'the enema should be reserved for women who have not had their bowels opened in the past 24 hours and have an obviously loaded rectum'.[7] The author of this study comments: 'Contamination after an enema was especially difficult to control, since it was more likely to be fluid.' This research was of particular interest as staff in the hospital where it was done were very unhappy about the project when it started and thought there would be mess everywhere. But they soon realized this was not so and that labour was much more pleasant for women when they did not have their bowels emptied artificially. As a result they surreptitiously omitted the enema or readily agreed with the woman when she demurred, so that the study had to be ended prematurely. Simply asking questions about procedures can start a process of change.

Immobilization

In many hospitals women in labour are put to bed. Yet women are more comfortable moving about during contractions and getting into positions in which they can lean forward. They spontaneously crouch, kneel or squat as labour advances and the birth approaches. The most uncomfortable position of all is lying down flat on your back, and there is evidence that it makes the first stage of labour longer and unnecessarily painful.[8] If a woman is lying on her back, with her legs either drawn up or suspended in the air with her feet in stirrups, she is not only uncomfortable but has to work much harder to push the baby out.

If you have anaesthesia, or anything but the smallest dose of pain-relieving drugs, there may be no alternative *but* to be in bed. One study of mobility in labour seemed to demonstrate conclusively that women do not want to leave their beds. This is hardly surprising, as in that hospital most women had already received large doses of pethidine and it would have been difficult for them to stand up, let alone walk about.[9]

If you decide that you don't want to be in bed all the time, you can prepare yourself for Active Birth, and some guidelines for this are on pp. 63–8.

Loss of privacy

In many hospitals the delivery room is a public arena and some labour wards are like a busy airport concourse or rail terminus. Even when each woman has her own labour room, there is often no privacy. People barge in and out without knocking, or if they do knock, do not wait for an answer. Doctors and nurses chat to each other about irrelevant topics or discuss the management of labour as if she were a log of wood. Sometimes attendants talk about a delivery that went badly wrong, or another particularly interesting case, in her presence and seem unaware that this can be terribly frightening.

If you would prefer an intimate atmosphere for your labour it may be a good idea to say in your birth plan that you would like as much peace and privacy as possible and to have continuity of care from just one or two nurses or midwives. You may find that dimming lights and playing music also helps.

Isolation

One element of transitional rituals in traditional societies – puberty rites for example – is separation of the novitiate from family and friends, from all the ordinary, everyday human relationships which have significance, and removal to a special place of isolation. In the twentieth century, until the mid-seventies, a woman having a baby in our Western culture was often similarly isolated from those closest to her. When she entered the hospital her husband was forced to leave her in professional hands and walked out with a suitcase of her clothes and personal belongings. She became merely another maternity case.

The introduction of husbands into the labour room changed all that, but this has still not come about in many countries, notably the USSR, where the father of the baby may not be allowed to step over the threshold of the hospital. After the birth he must stand in the street watching to see if by a sign through a window his wife can tell him whether they have had a girl or a boy.

The change came in the West partly because of the insistence of couples that they wanted to be together for this supremely important event in their lives. (One father, for example, given permission to be with his wife during labour, but not for delivery, handcuffed himself to the side of the delivery table.) It also happened because doctors began to see that when a woman had a companion with her she was calmer, needed fewer drugs for pain relief and was a more 'cooperative patient'. So the medical profession's acceptance of fathers in childbirth was double-edged. Some obstetricians quickly learnt that they could collude with a man to keep the woman obedient, talk 'science' together over her head, and persuade her to submit to interventions she did not really want. Threatening the woman that her partner would be sent away if they did not both conform to the rules was a method further ensuring patient compliance.

In the early days the man might be told to sit in a corner and not speak or move. Gradually, however, it was discovered that he could be of real assistance in giving both physical and emotional support and in helping out with nursing chores. The danger now is that the special intimacy between a couple can be exploited by professionals for whom management of the father has become as much a skill as management of the woman in labour. He may be directed, for example, to watch the electronic fetal monitor, to tell her when contractions are coming. For any man who is unsure of his role and lacks confidence in his ability to give the right emotional support, this can lead to his concentrating on machinery instead of keeping in touch with his partner's emotional experience. He has become part of the team – no longer on her side, representing her wishes and nurturing through his special understanding of her needs.

Though fathers are in the labour and delivery room now, and are here to stay, it is sometimes very much on the hospital's terms and with a carefully scripted part to play. Other members of the family and friends, on the other hand, are often still firmly barred from access. The mother may not be allowed another woman with her in labour, for example and, if she has the baby's father with her, may be denied the right to have any other support person as well.

Transfer to delivery room

In many hospitals a woman is still moved to another room for delivery. This often entails tremendous emotional upheaval and disorientation. She is under the stress of almost continuous contractions and suddenly her whole environment changes. Unless there are reasons why she needs to be in a specially equipped theatre for an operative delivery, this should not happen. It is now being realized that there is less risk of cross-infection and far less physical disturbance and emotional stress as she starts the second stage if each woman has her own private birth room in which she can labour and deliver.

The management of the second stage

Drapes and masks

These were originally introduced in the nineteenth century in an attempt to create a sterile environment for birth. In fact, bacteria are transferred by doctors and nurses on their hands and clothing, not by ordinary breathing and talking, and there is less infection when staff do not wear masks.[10] The wearing of masks is, says a leader in the *Lancet*, 'no more than an expensive ritual'.[11] One tremendous advantage when those who are caring for you do *not* wear masks is that you can see their faces and relate to them as individuals.

Cheer-leading and pushing to order

Cheer-leading in the second stage also has a ceremonial quality. It may make everyone feel good, because there is a sense of all being in it together and at last getting somewhere. It can seem that if only the mother would push harder and longer the baby's head would appear, so everyone present exhorts her to greater effort. They may tell her to hold her breath for 10, 15 or even 20 seconds – and count them out for her. She may be cajoled, bullied and threatened with a forceps delivery if she does not try harder. When she holds her breath for a really long time, goes red in the face and gasps with effort, she is likely to be praised and told that she is doing it right now. Dripping with sweat, eyes bulging, little blood vessels bursting in her cheeks and eyes, and falling back exhausted once each contraction is over, she struggles to obey the commands of her cheer-leaders and tackles the second stage of labour as if she were in a prize fight.

Telling a woman when and how to push, and encouraging her to work as hard as she can, is no new obstetric invention. It has been hallowed by time, and tends to be taken for granted as the only way of giving help in the second stage. Yet it has many disadvantages. It is not only that the woman feels desperate, as if the baby will never be born, or that she is left afterwards with aching muscles and a sore throat, as if she had a bad dose of flu. When she holds her breath for a long time – more than about six seconds – and simultaneously exerts effort, there are changes in her heart rate and blood pressure, and the oxygen content of the blood going through to the baby is reduced. As she deliberately holds her breath and pushes hard her blood pressure drops until she comes up for air and gasps, when it shoots up again. She may get dizzy and faint in much the same way as some people suffering from constipation do as they struggle to empty their bowels (the reason why heart attacks often occur in the lavatory). It is not surprising that if a woman strains like this for a long time – an hour or more – abnormalities in the baby's heart rate may be discovered. This practice has led to the conclusion that the second stage of labour is always dangerous for the baby, so that strict time-limits are set on it by obstetricians. It is not, however, the length of time itself but prolonged straining and breath-holding that put the baby at risk.

So this is another subject you may want to discuss in advance with your care-giver. Is any time-limit set on the second stage? If so, what is it? Will you be told to push or can you take the second stage at your own pace? In the process of discussing this you will realize that another question is raised: when is the second stage believed to start? It is one thing for a doctor to say, 'I don't like a baby's head to be too long on the perineum', and quite another to say that you only have an hour from full dilatation of the cervix before you must be at the point of delivery. The second stage is sometimes considered to be the whole process following full dilatation until delivery of the baby. It is much more in line with physiology to consider it as the time during which you are pushing spontaneously. Since a woman does not get an overwhelming urge to push until the baby's head is on the perineum, this means that there is often a lull following full dilatation during which she is not doing anything deliberate to push the baby out and responds to the contractions very much as if they were first-stage ones – that is, breathing and relaxing with them. However, another ceremony which has become an integral part of childbirth is to urge the woman to push at this point – 'because', she is often told, 'the baby is just sitting there waiting to be born'. If she says she does not want to yet, she may be coaxed into trying and persuaded to hold her breath. She often feels bewildered by this and also worried that her body is not working correctly. She may feel rather like a little girl sitting on her potty unable to produce.

When a woman starts pushing before her body is ready for it she

(a) Front view

(b) Side view

13 The baby's journey through the pelvis: how the stations are numbered.

may tire herself out by the time she can really work with her uterus to press the baby through the birth canal. Moreover she pushes ineffectively because there is no urge to show her exactly when and for how long each push should last and how strong it should be. She may feel guilty and disheartened by this.

In order to be born, the baby's head comes down through different levels of the pelvis which are called 'stations'. These are identified by numbers from minus 5, which means that the top of the baby's head is 5 centimetres above the ischial spines (small bits of the pelvis which project into the sides of the pelvic cavity), through zero, where the head is level with the ischial spines, and on down through plus 1 to plus 5, the position at birth.

If by the time the cervix is completely dilated the head is already low, the pushing urge comes at or around full dilatation. When the baby's head is high there is no spontaneous desire to push. In fact, contractions often get weak and far apart, or may cease entirely for about 20 minutes – sometimes longer. This is a marvellous opportunity to have a rest and get refreshed in preparation for the active second stage. Having your hair brushed or a luxurious back massage, taking a shower, strolling around and breathing some fresh air are all good things to do during this interval. This lull has been called 'the latent phase of the second stage', and corresponds to the gentle lead-in to labour which many women have at the beginning of the first stage.[12] It is only when the head comes down through the cervix on to perineal tissues that contractions will build up again, when what is known as 'Fergusson's reflex' is established. (It is a fair bet that Fergusson, who was a man, never felt it, but as with many other female physiological functions, a man's name is attached to it.)

Getting a baby born is not only a matter of achieving full dilatation. Tissues in and around the birth canal and the perineum need to open up before the baby can be pressed through the vagina without injury to the mother. Full dilatation of the cervix precedes this further dilatation. Forcing the baby down through a rigid passage is difficult for the mother and can be hard on the baby too. A British professor of obstetrics states categorically: 'It is a serious fault to force delivery merely because a set time has elapsed on the clock. Women must not be urged to commence bearing down merely because the cervix is fully dilated.'[13]

When she pushes because she is being told she must, or because she feels she ought to, the mother's blood pressure sometimes goes up and there are 'late decelerations' of the fetal heart. This means that the heart rate gets slower at the end of a contraction and remains slow after it has finished. A forceps delivery is then performed because of fetal and/or maternal distress.

All this can be avoided if a woman is allowed to take her own time. Labour should not be a competition to see how quickly it can be over. It is not only a question of being able to find your own rhythm once you are in the second stage, but also of being able to enjoy the rest period which often comes after full dilatation, waiting to push until *you* want to and until it is impossible to ask whether you should or should not, because that is the only thing you *can* do!

Some women want to push *before* they are fully dilated. The custom then is to instruct them not to push, and if they cannot obey anaesthesia may be given at this point, in case forceful pushing produces trauma to the cervix. A premature urge to push often occurs if the baby is occipito-posterior (facing forward). Ordering a woman not to push when she finds it unavoidable causes anxiety, especially if there is nothing that she can do instead. A change of position, leaning forward or being on all fours, is a more effective way of helping. But, in fact, research has failed to show that there is any harm in gentle pushing before the cervix is fully dilated. Pushing like this is quite different from the kind of pushing that starts when a woman is in a state of panic because she has been told not to.

Commands to push or not to push are another way in which ritual intrudes on a woman's trust in her own body, often causing anxiety and distress.

Management of the third stage

The time from delivery of the baby until the delivery of the placenta and membranes constitutes the third stage of labour. As soon as the baby is born the placenta starts to separate naturally from the inner lining of the uterus. This happens because the uterus continues to contract, and since the placenta cannot contract it is automatically peeled off. The placenta is attached to the wall of the uterus rather as a postage stamp might be stuck on stretched elastic. If you let the elastic spring back the stamp would automatically peel away.

But this process can be delayed by things done at the birth and immediately afterwards. The first intervention that can cause problems is the simple act of clamping the cord while blood is still pulsating through it.[14] Until the seventeenth century the cord was simply cut, not clamped. But when doctors began to take over from midwives, and as women began to give birth in bed, rather than on birth stools, the practice of cord-clamping was introduced in order to avoid soiling the bed-linen. When blood cannot drain through the cord, the placenta becomes solid and compact like a firmly packed cushion, a blood clot forms behind it where the blood cannot flow and it sometimes gets stuck.

So doctors began to pull on the cord in order to get the placenta out before the cervix closed up, and taught midwives to do this too. If it is done before the placenta has fully separated blood oozes from partially torn blood vessels. As a result there is greater blood loss than if everything was left to happen naturally, and sometimes the placenta is retained while at the same time the woman is haemorrhaging.

Then in the thirties ergometrine, an alkaloid of a fungus that grows on rye, was introduced to make the uterus contract harder. This entailed getting the placenta out more quickly still, in case it became trapped inside the firmly contracted uterus. Since then other oxytocic drugs have been developed, combined with ergometrine or alone, and their use is now standard practice in obstetrics. An injection is given in the mother's thigh to force the uterus to contract as soon as the baby's anterior shoulder is delivered, or immediately following the birth. Then the cord is clamped to avoid large amounts of excess blood being forced into the baby's circulation by these abnormally strong contractions. This is followed by 'controlled cord traction' to pull out the placenta before the cervix closes up.

All this is done to avoid post-partum haemorrhage (PPH). Pools of blood are formed when finger-like projections all over the maternal side of the placenta are sheered away, but if the placenta is expelled quickly the uterus can clamp down on itself, so that there is minimal blood loss. The drugs employed are useful, and can be life-saving if there is heavy bleeding, but there are disadvantages with their routine use, as there is also with early cord-clamping and pulling on the cord:

- When the cord is clamped while still pulsating the baby is cut off from its oxygen supply and thrown on to its own resources. There must be no delay in the start of breathing.
- Early cord-clamping also deprives the baby of blood which is rightly its own. It is especially important for a premature baby to receive this blood.
- The third stage tends to last longer when the cord is clamped while blood is still pulsating through it. The placenta usually separates easily if it is allowed to bleed.[15]
- Ergometrine causes a rise in the mother's blood pressure and can result in headaches, dizziness, ringing in the ears, palpitations and cramp in the legs and back. It makes any nausea and vomiting much worse.
- Once ergometrine has been given, if the clamping of the cord is left

for as long as three minutes the baby gets half as much blood again as if there were no intervention. One result of this is that many babies develop jaundice because they have more red cells than they can cope with.

- When the cord is pulled it sometimes breaks accidentally. Occasionally, too, when part of the placenta is still attached, a bit gets left behind. If part or all of the placenta gets trapped in the contracted uterus, there must be manual removal under general anaesthesia. If it has not separated the uterus is occasionally even pulled inside out.

- For a woman who is rhesus negative with a rhesus positive baby there is a special disadvantage in these procedures. As the placenta is peeling off, some blood cells can escape into her circulation. This is more likely to happen when the cord is clamped early, because a good deal of the baby's blood is in the placenta at that stage, and as pressure rises in the placenta some blood vessels may burst. This results in iso-immunization (the build up of antibodies in her bloodstream), which can jeopardize the next pregnancy.[16]

If you want to have a natural third stage you can ask:

- To be in an upright position (squatting or kneeling) for delivery of the placenta, so that gravity helps its expulsion.
- Not to be given ergometrine or any form of oxytocin unless you start to bleed heavily.
- Not to have the cord clamped until it has stopped pulsating.
- To deliver the placenta yourself by pushing.

Remember, though, that if an injection to make the uterus contract *is* given, the cord *should* be clamped to avoid the baby receiving too much blood.

How the baby is treated

Handling of delivery

How would you react if told there was a species of animal which hung its young upside down at birth and hit it? That used to be the practice when a baby was born, and there are doubtless some doctors who still do it. The standard TV scene of delivery shows a doctor suspending a screaming baby from its heels as he announces through his mask, 'It's a boy!' This practice is unnecessary and may be harmful. Frederick Leboyer claims that sudden extension of the spine after being curled up in the uterus could be painful and shocking for the baby, and may cause physical harm: 'The spinal column has been strained, bent, pushed, and twisted to the limits of its endurance – and now it is robbed of all support. And the head, so supremely involved in the passage outward – now it also is dangling, twisting. And this at the very moment when, in order to calm this vast terror, this panic, what is essential is a coming together with the mother, a *reuniting*.'[17]

At birth the baby encounters cold air and noise of a very different kind from that experienced in the uterus, is placed in unfamiliar contact with cloth, metal and plastic and put under bright light for the first time. It is a dramatic transition from the warmth, comfort, glowing light and velvety softness of the uterus. Hands touch the baby, sometimes roughly as if the child were a lump of meat, sometimes tenderly, expressing reverence for the new life.

You may want to think about the environment into which the baby is born and the way in which your child is welcomed to life. You can ask, for example, that the birth take place in a dimly lit room, that the voices of attendants should be lowered and there should be no extraneous sounds, that the baby should be delivered straight on to your abdomen and that you can be in skin-to-skin contact for as long as you choose. When the birth is straightforward it is often possible for you to lift the baby from your body yourself, especially if you have help and encouragement to do so. That is an incredible experience!

Eyedrops

In some countries the baby must receive eyedrops as prophylaxis against gonococcal blindness. Silver nitrate treatment was introduced in Germany by Crede in the nineteenth century and is still often used, though there are today better alternatives which do not irritate the eye – tetracycline and erythromycine, which may be even more effective.[18] In some countries, for example the United Kingdom, eye treatment for newborn babies has been discarded unless it is shown to be needed. If you are having a baby outside the UK this may be another issue which you want to consider, perhaps discuss with a paediatrician and include in your birth plans.

Bonding time

A new rite has been added to the care of the newborn in hospital – 'bonding time'. In theory it is a marvellous idea and acknowledges a new concern about the relationship between mother and baby and the need for midwives and doctors to understand emotional aspects of the post-partum experience. In practice it becomes another ceremonial procedure.

Feeling you have to bond in ten minutes flat (or knowing that people are watching you to see if you are bonding correctly) is unlikely to help you fall in love with your baby. It is more difficult still if the baby is carted off to the nursery. Even having the baby close to your bed but being told not to 'disturb' it interferes with spontaneous behaviour and emotions. In many new mothers' experience it is best to be free to cuddle the baby whenever you want, have lengthy sucking sessions in which you ignore time and just enjoy being together, and have the baby in bed whenever and for as long as you choose.

Many women do not fall in love with their babies immediately. You may need time to be close to your baby and to get to know each other. As you think ahead to the hours and days after birth, consider what is likely to help you most to relax and enjoy your baby.

On the other hand, you may also want to know that someone will keep an eye on the baby if you wish to sleep and find it difficult to drop off if the baby is in your bed, as some women do, or you may feel that you simply must have a night's more or less undisturbed sleep and need to know there is someone there to care for the baby if you decide to do this.

You will get more ideas about how you would like those days after birth to be if you talk to other new mothers and find out how it was for them. Whether or not you are planning to breastfeed your baby, and that is undoubtedly the best start to life for any baby, you may find it helpful to read another book of mine, *The Experience of Breastfeeding* (Penguin).

Incorporate your wishes for after the birth in your birth plan. Remember to be flexible and think what you might want if you are very tired, or uncomfortable with stitches in your perineum. Whatever happens, you will then have prepared for your baby's first days of life outside your body with forethought and understanding.

Autonomous Birth

18

THE CONCEPT OF AUTONOMY

AUTONOMY: Freedom ... Liberty ... Scope ... Self-determination ...
Non-interference ... Emancipation
AUTONOMOUS: Independent ... Unconstrained ... Unconfined ...
Unhindered ... Unshackled

Roget's Thesaurus

The most important distinction between styles of birth is that between *obstetrically managed* birth and *autonomous* birth. Before you start to draw up your birth plan you need to consider which of these overall styles of childbirth you prefer. By 'autonomous' I mean that you make your own informed decisions between alternatives and give birth in an environment where you have the self-confidence to act spontaneously. You may need a great deal of help from other people to do this. Or you may have everything within yourself to give birth using your own power and energy.

The term 'natural childbirth' often implies a labour and delivery without intervention of any kind. Sometimes, however, intervention is helpful and is safer for the baby or results in a more positive birth experience for the mother. An autonomous birth is one in which the woman is free to do exactly what she feels like doing, including moving about – or lying down, if that is what she wants at the time – and in which she decides what help she needs. It is not only a matter of 'active birth' and being able to move about – though that is important – but of being an active birth-giver rather than a passive patient. It is basically a question of who accepts the main responsibility, and ultimately with whom the power lies – the obstetrician or you. Whether labour turns out to be natural or assisted, straightforward or complicated, short or long, and with or without pain-relieving drugs, when it is an event for which a woman accepts personal responsibility, considers the advantages and disadvantages of different alternatives, comes to her own decisions and has the freedom to follow them through, it is an autonomous experience.

Autonomous birth is not just a matter of writing down how you would like your birth to be, or not having people do things to you against your will. It is something much more positive than that. Autonomous birth entails:

- Choosing an environment for birth in which you are free to be yourself. You can forget your public, polite, 'performing' self and surrender to intensity of feeling. You prepare yourself as fully as you can to meet the stresses and challenges of childbirth and to ride the waves of a powerful and fathomless experience.
- Being able to rely on continuing companionship in labour from someone of your choice who in no way represents or reinforces the power of the hospital, but is there to support *you* and can be your anchor in a stormy sea.
- Having a midwife or doctor who understands what you are trying to do and who knows how to give positive support. Some professionals do not realize that if you hope to manage without drugs or any other intervention in labour it is not enough simply to leave you alone to 'get on with it'. You need positive support for what you are doing. If labour is long or tiring, or you hit a storm in the late first stage, or if there is a hold-up at any phase, you will need other kinds of help: warm encouragement, emotional support, suggestions about ways in which you can deal with the challenges yourself (such as help with breathing and relaxation, walking about, taking a hot shower or relaxing in the bath, being massaged where you have pain or there are signs of tension, kissing and cuddling and nipple stimulation from someone you love, to stimulate your uterus).
- Having the information you need in order to weigh up the pros and cons of different courses of action and learning how to use obstetricians and other professionals as valuable resource people. This is far from straightforward, since access to information is controlled by those in power, and the very act of seeking knowledge is seen by some doctors as threatening. Yet one thing is clear: 'If you don't know your options, you don't have any.'[1]
- Speaking and acting with assurance so that your wishes are clearly understood and you define the limits of what other people do to you. As we have seen already, in Chapter 10, it is not easy to be assertive in childbirth unless you have developed the habit of calm, confident assertion in general life. For many women labour is an

overwhelming experience in which they feel swept along by forces beyond their control. This is why, however much knowledge you have about alternatives, and however sure of yourself you feel during pregnancy, assertiveness should not be left to chance and you need to practise and cultivate it during pregnancy.

- Having the strength that comes from flexibility and awareness of the alternatives in any situation you are likely to encounter, and avoiding the weakness inherent in rigidity.

> Consider the different elements of autonomous birth as I have outlined them in this list, and if this is the kind of birth you want, use it to assess your own strengths in preparing for such an experience. Make a note of each of your strong points.
>
> Then look over the list again to see where you need to do more work and perhaps seek help to prepare yourself for autonomous birth. Note any decisions you want to take as a result of this.

Autonomous birth is not necessarily easy, straightforward or brief. Jan's labour, for instance, was at times stormy and frustrating. But she was clear in her mind about what she wanted and approached the whole experience with verve, had loving care from her partner and women friends and, with enlightened support from her midwives, succeeded in having an autonomous birth.

In the early phases she was so excited that she over-reacted to the initial signs of labour and expected the baby to be born almost any minute. She phoned me and asked if I thought she should go into hospital yet. I urged her to stay at home, see friends, go for walks, eat when she was hungry and keep moving. However, this latent phase of labour, during which contractions became increasingly painful, lasted close on eight hours. She remained keyed up and too alert to rest properly. Her husband rang me and said, 'She is exhausting herself with her own determination.' Here is Jan's own description of what happened:

> The atmosphere in the house truly felt festive – like we were getting ready for a special event. P and I walked down to the super-market – good, brisk walk with contractions coming every five minutes. Then we had dinner of rich chicken broth, wholewheat bread – contractions still maintaining the same intensity, lasting 40 to 45 seconds every five to six minutes. From 9 p.m. to 11.30 or 12 could

manage the contractions by holding on to the mantelpiece and rocking. Also walked around the house frequently. Around 12 started to hang from Bill's shoulders – bend at the knees and sway from foot to foot. That as it turns out was going to be my most enduring and comfortable position.

I *nicely* insisted that I wear my own blue cotton shirt, not regulation gown. We went to the big Active Birth Room – good atmosphere. When given an internal I was only three to four centimetres dilated ... The midwife who admitted me put a fetal heart monitor on – seemed alarmed by a sudden fall in heart-beat – put an oxygen mask on me. Bill annoyed, as it was the machine's fault and should not have been a cause of worry for us.

I managed to doze off between contractions. Bill sat in front of me while Cathy rubbed my lower back – felt good. To my great happiness the lovely midwife who shared the parentcraft class – Heather – was our midwife. Couldn't have been better. Started suggesting alternative positions for dealing with contractions – on all fours – raising the height of the bed so that I could lean on pillows – birthing stool. I was still finding that hanging from Bill's shoulders was the best way to deal with the contractions.

Starting to say 'Oh God!' a lot of the time.

At 10.30 Heather suggested a shower. Cathy talked me through the next half-hour in the shower. During a contraction I held on to a vertical bar and literally belly-danced, trying to relax my rectum and allow the head to drop, dilating the cervix. Between contractions I sat on a bench, dropped my head, attempted to let everything go limp while Cathy sprayed me with water. I was so relaxed on occasions that I would fall asleep, only waking because another contraction was coming.

Bill was lying on the bed, the midwife was sitting chatting to him and a young student nurse, all very jolly. The contractions were tough. I remember saying to Cathy, towards the end of the shower, 'I physically can't take much more, I am just so tired.'

But when I returned to the room the urge to push came. The energy was unbelievable. Heather did another internal and confirmed that I was about nine centimetres and yes, I could start pushing. Hallelujah! What a turnabout in my energies! I became euphoric – remember loading film in the camera between contractions, tried several different positions – on all fours, but didn't find this to be as successful as sitting in a very vertical position or squatting on the bed with arms around the shoulders of midwife and student nurse.

The pushing sensation is a most extraordinary one – the whole universe being pushed into the rectum. The sun was shining brightly into the room. I felt a cocoon of support around me. The pushes were strong. Never needless chatter. Episiotomy was discussed, with the unanimous decision to avoid it if possible – meant twice panting like a frenzied dog in spite of the fact that the uterus continued to push.

When Heather said to feel the head the emotion building up in me was like a volcano about to erupt. Once the head and shoulders had emerged I pulled him up on to me. I remember very well the tears of joy and relief and disbelief as he lay on my chest – me fumbling with a breast which he was not at all interested in. He cried immediately but soon stopped.

I had a small lateral vaginal tear. An experienced doctor handled it beautifully while I cuddled William. Then he and I just lay together for a while, and Heather brought me in toast and tea.

The euphoric feeling was with both Bill and me and we only had to look at each other or the baby and we'd start to cry.

Plans often need adapting in the light of experience. But this need not deprive you of autonomy.

Tricia, for example, very much wanted to have her second baby at home. Following a Caesarean delivery, first time round, however, her doctor was unhappy with the suggestion, but keen that she should have a natural birth if possible. 'After a great deal of thought, discussion and soul-searching,' Tricia explained to me, 'we decided to have the baby in hospital. We felt happy with this decision because we were very fortunate to find an excellent obstetrician who feels as we do, that birth is a normal, natural process, which should not be interfered with unless there are very strong indications for doing so. She thought our requests for no electronic monitoring, no ARM [artificial rupture of membranes], no episiotomy and no Syntometrine [an injection to help expel the placenta] were perfectly understandable.' This is how Tricia's labour went:

After two false labours, I went into labour proper at 5 a.m. My husband stayed off work and we had a lovely morning playing with our daughter, walking the dog and shopping. At 12 noon the contractions began to demand my relaxation and attention. By 2 p.m. I felt the need to breathe through them. By 4.30 p.m. I had to do upper-chest breathing and occasionally had to disappear into the bedroom with my husband to regain control over the contractions by relaxation and breathing. Fortunately my mother was here to play with my daughter, so my husband was able to give me his full attention, without which I could not have coped.

By 8.30 p.m. I was only four centimetres dilated and the contractions had been coming at intervals of two minutes – lasting for one minute – for some time. I was beginning to feel that I might not be able to manage if I had many hours to go. At 9.30 p.m. I asked my husband to phone the hospital and inform them that we were going in. As he put the phone down I began to shake and feel sick. I knew that these were signs of transition, but didn't dare hope that I was so far on.

The half-hour car journey was very trying, but once in the delivery room I was sick, which gave me enormous relief. They asked Michael what we did and didn't want, and put a mattress on the floor for us. I suddenly heard myself grunting and felt frightened that they would tell me I couldn't push yet. I felt then that I would lose control. Much to my relief, they told me to push, and they ruptured the membranes.

We had wanted some pictures of the delivery but I was unable to let my husband go to take them, so the paediatrician kindly took over this role. After a couple of contractions when I felt quite confused I got into the rhythm of pushing. The midwife went out of her way to avoid doing an episiotomy. I had a quick second stage of 20 minutes and Sophie was delivered at 11.06 p.m.

I enjoyed my labour and delivery enormously. In fact it was the best day of my life. It was the most fulfilling thing I have ever done.

I feel that I have held the universe in my hands.

19

DRAWING UP YOUR BIRTH PLAN

One way of helping yourself towards autonomy in childbirth is to construct a birth plan based on all the notes you have already made as you have gone through this book. It will give those caring for you a clear signal as to what you want and provide a good basis for discussion.

When you get down to writing your plan, here are some general guidelines:

At the beginning of your plan there should be a brief outline of principles relating to *behaviour*, not attitudes. You can't change people's attitudes, but you can monitor what they do. You might want to say, for example, 'Except in an emergency, if intervention of any kind is proposed, I want to be told what it is, its effects and side-effects and why it is considered necessary, and have time to discuss this with my partner in private.' Or you can say, 'For me, effective pain relief by whatever means are available is of primary importance,' or, 'I want to be certain that the person who cares for me in labour is someone with whom I have already established a relationship.'

The birth plan should go on to list particular requests. Emphasize the positive rather than simply saying that you don't want something. For instance, 'No episiotomy!' sounds like part of a manifesto. It may make the doctor or midwife anxious about what to do if there is stress on your perineum and you are about to tear. It is better to say: 'I should prefer a tear to an episiotomy, and hope to be able to deliver slowly to avoid any perineal wound.'

If you are having your baby in an American hospital, make sure that your plan covers everything that happens from the time you are admitted. There are problems with birth plans in some hospitals because they have a system of 'standing orders'. This means that when a woman is admitted, labour is conducted according to a protocol which is applied to all patients of that doctor or nurse-midwife, or sometimes to all patients in the hospital. This may be quite different from the things she has

negotiated. You can ask in advance whether standard care is provided until your own doctor arrives, and make an arrangement with him or her and with the head nurse to ensure your wishes are respected from the moment you go into hospital.

Your plan should not be vague. 'I want an active birth' may leave someone who is uninformed not able to understand what you are planning. Be clear and specific: e.g., 'I wish to be free to be out of bed and move around throughout labour.'

Show that you are aware that in labour you may want something different from what you envisaged in pregnancy: e.g., 'I want to be able to eat during labour, if I feel like it at the time.'

Your plan should take into account the care you would like to have if there are deviations from the normal: e.g., 'I am happy to have electronic fetal monitoring if labour is prolonged, the baby is in an unusual position or there are deviations from the normal which are fully explained to me. Otherwise I should like to have intermittent monitoring.'

Think of building your birth plan in several stages. To begin with, set down the things which are most important to you, together with any interventions you particularly want to avoid. This should be followed by discussion with your doctor or midwife. You will then want to find out more about certain aspects of care and procedures about which you have not already made up your mind, so you will need a period of discussion with other women who have had babies, reading, and so on. By 36 weeks you should have a clear idea of what you want and of your priorities. Talk it over freely with the person who is going to be your birth companion. Then draw up a new, modified birth plan and discuss this at one of your prenatal visits. You can ask your care-giver to confirm on the final version that you have talked together about these subjects. One copy should go in your notes, and you should have another with you in labour. Then there can be no confusion.

Bear in mind that doctors and midwives are very anxious about birth plans. You may find you need to reassure them about why you want a birth plan. Explain that you are flexible and will accept intervention if you consider it necessary, and that you are glad to have advice (even though sometimes in the end your conclusion may be different from theirs).

Here are some examples of birth plans drawn up by real women – not models on which to base your own. First a short simple one:

TO THE MIDWIFE WHO ATTENDS ME IN LABOUR

If my labour proceeds in a spontaneous and natural manner with no complications, then the following points are of main concern to me. It will help me to relax more if I feel they can be taken into consideration:

1. If possible, could my baby be born in a room where the lights can be dimmed after delivery.

2. Unless it is absolutely necessary, I would prefer not to be continually monitored by machinery which prohibits my movement.

3. Because I worry about their effect on the baby, could drugs not be administered unless they are requested by me.

4. If I am not too exhausted after delivery and the baby is fine, could the baby be placed on me. Also, could the cord not be clamped until it has stopped pulsating unless there is a specific reason for doing so.

5. After delivery and provided all is well, I would like to keep my baby with me in order to breastfeed on demand and I would be grateful for any help or advice from staff.

The following birth plan is in the form of suggestions for a woman to consider. It is used at McMaster University Hospital, Hamilton, Ontario:

It is always helpful to give some thought in advance to your baby's birth, and to your stay in hospital. Putting your plans in writing will help you to clarify them in your own mind and will allow us to discuss them with you.

PREGNANCY

Are you taking (or have you taken) any childbirth education classes? The hospital maternity tour? If not, do you plan to take any?

LABOR AND BIRTH

(a) *If all goes normally* (Please make note of anything that may be important to you, such as who you might wish to have with you, your plans in regard to medication, epidural, place or position for birth, etc.)

(b) *Contingency plans* (Please note your thoughts about what you might want done if things don't go the way you planned; if, for example, you have a long or difficult labor, require more pain relief than you had anticipated, need forceps, episiotomy or a Caesarean; if the baby is premature or ill. It is often valuable to think about things like this in advance.)

(c) *Personal plans* (Do you wish to take photos, bring in a tape recorder for music, or do you have any special requests to bring to our attention?)

POST PARTUM

(Any special plans about baby feeding, or baby care?)

FOR OUR INFORMATION

Who will be the doctor for the baby in hospital?
If you have a boy, do you wish him to be circumcised?
Do you plan on early discharge from hospital?
Thank you. This sheet will be kept with your chart, and will serve as a guide to those who will be caring for you in hospital.

A problem with hospital-designed birth plans, however, is that they define your parameters of choice. They are like set menus. They are very useful in getting women, some of whom might not have thought beforehand about what they wanted, or did not know that there were any alternatives, to make decisions about the kind of care they prefer. But they may have the effect of actually preventing some alternatives ever being considered. So if hospitals do devise their own birth plans, it is important that they discuss and develop them with women having babies, preferably through some kind of study group in which there can be a free exchange of ideas with the staff.

The next birth plan is a sample one devised by the women's consumer health organization Choice in Philadelphia:

We have written this birth plan in partnership with our midwife so that we can be involved in the birth of our baby. This is an ideal plan, based on our hope that labor and birth will be normal and that Joanna and the baby will not have problems. We know that there may be problems or emergencies, and that we may need to use a medication or procedure we would rather avoid. If this happens, we would like to have the problem explained and our questions answered, so that we can give our informed consent.

As long as there are no problems with Joanna's or the baby's health:

1 Paul, the baby's father, would like to be present during labor and birth.
2. Joanna would rather not be shaved or have an enema.
3. She would rather not have an IV inserted unless labor is very long, or medication is needed.
4. Joanna and Paul have learned breathing and relaxation exercises. If it is needed, she would prefer to use a mild medication to ease the pain before using anesthesia. We would like to avoid general anesthesia.
5. As long as she is comfortable, she would like to walk or sit during labor.
6. If labor contractions are not strong enough, we would like to strengthen them by doing these things if possible: walking, taking a warm shower, then, if necessary, amniotomy, and uterine stimulation only if essential.
7. We would like to have our baby's heart monitored by the midwife using a fetoscope, and contractions monitored by the midwife listening to Joanna's description of them and feeling her abdomen to tell their strength and length.

If it is needed, we would rather use external than internal electronic monitoring.

8. Joanna would like to give birth in the same room she labors in, in a position that is comfortable for her.
9. If possible she would like to avoid an episiotomy.
10. After the baby is born, we would like to have one to two hours with her to hold her, nurse her and get to know each other. If there is a problem with the baby's health and she must go to the nursery right away, Paul would like to go with her and Joanna would like to join them when she can.
11. If a Cesarean birth is needed we would rather use regional anesthesia, and Paul would like to be in the delivery room. If possible we would like to spend time together before the baby is sent to the nursery.
12. While Joanna and the baby are in the hospital we would like the baby to room-in so that she can feed her whenever she is hungry.

We look forward to working with you during labor and the birth of our baby.

Joanna Adamson
Paul Adamson

I agree to honor the wishes of Joanna and Paul as long as labor is normal and the mother and baby's health allows it. If a problem comes up, I will discuss it with them before taking the necessary medical steps.

Susan Brown, CNM

As you see, the advantage of this one is that it is signed by the care-giver, in this case the nurse-midwife. Like other birth plans, it is not a legal contract, but when plans are signed in this way it gives them a certain formal status which suggests that they are morally binding.

It is sometimes asserted that birth plans do not 'work', and never can, because doctors control the strings of power. It is true that in the last resort a woman may be coerced into compliance with care-givers who do not respect her right to make decisions. But birth plans can be a valuable way of opening negotiation with care-givers, building communication – and, indeed, of educating them about what women want. It is through such ventures, through pressure put on the medical system primarily from outside, rather than from changes doctors and midwives themselves introduce, that childbirth can be improved for *all* women, not only those who are vocal and know what they are seeking.

You may be surprised by your care-giver's readiness to cooperate with your birth plans, even in a hospital which a few years back was not open to suggestions from patients. Kathy, for example, told me that she was very unsure about how her birth plan would be received in a hospital in the American Mid-West which was not known for being progressive.

She was pleased when she was invited to go on a tour of the labour and postnatal wards and encouraged to ask as many questions as she wanted: 'A senior nurse said that they might be introducing a pro-forma birth plan to be issued at the first prenatal visit – not to impose anything on the mother but to give her something to think about, if she wanted to.' When Kathy met the head nurse she produced her birth plan, but the head nurse seemed 'rather put out that I had felt it necessary to put my wishes in writing, since most of what I had asked for was standard practice'. Here is Kathy's birth plan:

I would like the birth of our baby to be as natural as possible, as long as the life and well-being of me and the baby are not endangered.

Enema	No.
Shaving	No.
Artificial breaking of waters	Only if necessary: please discuss first.
Induction	Only if necessary: please discuss and check dilatation first.
Electronic fetal monitoring	Internal: preferably only in the event of an epidural. External: not continuously. Monitoring for a few minutes at a time every half-hour (say) would be perfectly acceptable.
Position	As I feel the need at the time. I am likely to want to move around, at least in the early stages.
Pain relief	None if I can manage without. If Demerol [pethidine] is used, please start with 50 mg, and check dilatation first. Epidural only after discussion.
Episiotomy	I would rather matters went slowly enough for this not to be necessary. I would prefer to tear rather than be cut. Please discuss first.
Delivery of baby	On to my stomach immediately. I would like the baby to be able to suckle if it wants.
Cutting the cord	Not until it has stopped pulsating (at the earliest).
Pitocin [Syntometrine] injection	If this can be avoided, so much the better, otherwise not until the cord is cut.
Aspiration of mucus	If the baby is breathing satisfactorily, then no aspiration please.
Environment	At delivery or before, lights dimmed; no unnecessary noises please.

Section	If time, then epidural; I realize that a general anesthetic may be necessary. I would like a trial of labor first, please. To the best of my knowledge I am not allergic to penicillin.
Feeding	Breastfeeding only, on demand both day and night.

My husband Dave knows and is thoroughly familiar with the contents of this birth plan; he will be able to discuss any aspects as required if I am not in a fit state to do so!

As it turned out, Kathy didn't get all the things she asked for in her birth plan, but the relationship with her care-givers was so good and discussion so open that from her point of view the birth went exactly as she wished. This is how she described labour:

At 5 a.m. I woke to find myself leaking. At 6.30 a.m. contractions started and seemed to me to be very close – closer than I had expected so early on – about three to four minutes – deep breathing and concentrating on the rest of me helped – especially shoulders and legs. I went into hospital and was examined – two centimetres.

I was put on an external monitor for half an hour. The nurse brought me some toast, tea and marmalade. I managed half a slice and half a cup, but no more. Somewhere around this time my body demonstrated its lack of need for an enema by emptying itself from both ends, so I made no further attempt to eat any breakfast.

I sipped water using a straw – a godsend. I couldn't hold a cup – Dave had to for me. I remember hearing music vaguely – Haydn, Vivaldi. I rocked back and forth through these contractions – I really felt I could not move about but this small movement helped. I asked for Demerol at 9.45. When they examined me they said that as I was eight centimetres dilated perhaps I could manage without it. This news bucked me tremendously. Sometimes I forgot to breathe in between contractions. Dave realized and reminded me. I remember trying to work out my rate of dilatation per hour given that I'd gone from two to eight centimetres in three hours, to give me some idea of how long it would take to get to ten centimetres. But I gave up.

When I said I was getting a different feeling, like pushing, people seemed to turn up rather suddenly. The midwife examined me and said I was 9½ centimetres and that there was a lip which was swelling. She suggested that I should turn over and stick my bottom in the air to drop the baby back and allow full dilatation, but it seemed too much of an effort, so she said she'd try something first, and on the next contraction she flipped the lip over the head and we were straight into the second stage at around 11 a.m. Dave helped me to get up and squat. I leaned forward on to my hands. I tried hanging on to Dave around his neck, but it didn't work so well, so I reverted to all fours. I began breathing too hard between contractions, and when the midwife queried whether I was still having a contraction, I calmed down. The pain of the contractions had gone. Instead there was the pain of stretching skin. At one point I said, 'It hurts,' and Dave said, 'It's got to,' and so I carried on.

The midwife, when she could feel the head coming, asked me to sit back so she would have more control. Dave was on my right, helping me to push from that side, and I held a lever on the left. At first they wanted little pushes, which Dave translated into terms I could cope with, in a rhythm – push, relax, push, relax. Then panting, then back to push, relax. Then, 'You can feel the head if you like. Do you want a mirror?' 'No thank you.' What an extraordinary feeling, to touch the head! In between contractions I could relax totally, and the sitting-back position, knees up, helped. It took several contractions to deliver the head. What a relief then! The stretching eased dramatically. Then some more for the shoulders, and suddenly I let go and the baby was on my stomach. Time: 11.25 a.m.

The cord stopped pulsating very soon and then they clamped it. For the delivery of the placenta I should have got up again and squatted, and not been in such a hurry, perhaps; but I didn't want to leave it too long so we agreed that I should have a pitocin injection and the placenta came away soon after. I had first degree tears to the labia and inside; the midwife thought I might get away with no stitches, but called the doctor anyway who decided to stitch, to guarantee a clean mend.

Afterwards the midwife commented on how relaxed I'd been and this had undoubtedly helped the birth and minimized the tearing. The baby's head was apparently rather big.

At 1 p.m. we returned to my room. How strange! The last time I was in that elevator I was carrying Blob. Now I was carrying Michael.

Look back at Kathy's birth plan. Nearly everything was just as she wanted. Though she asked for Demerol once she was having strong contractions, the midwife, realizing that she wanted as natural a birth as possible, encouraged her to cope without it by letting her know how fast she was dilating. Kathy had asked for a few minutes of electronic monitoring every half hour or so. In fact, her midwife thought it was better to do continuous monitoring for half an hour early in labour to make sure that all was well, and then to monitor the baby's heart using a fetal stethoscope which did not involve any electronics at all. To avoid an episiotomy the midwife worked closely and carefully with her so that birth could be slow and gentle. She had a uterine stimulant after the cord was cut because she was impatient to deliver the placenta, but this was only done after discussion and with her agreement. Kathy feels that her birth plan worked well.

One of the great criticisms of birth plans is that a woman may set her sights on an ideal and be very shocked if labour is difficult or there are complications. This is why it is important also to make contingency plans to cope with the unexpected. Julie and Philip had decided on a home birth and Julie's sister, Penny, who is a midwife, was looking forward to caring for her in labour. In the event, the baby was breech and after talking it over they decided that it would be safer to have the baby in a hospital where there was an intensive care neonatal unit. So she rewrote her birth plan in this way:

BIRTH PLAN

We are obviously disappointed at not being able to have the home birth that we had planned, but we recognise that hospital is the safest place to have a breech birth. The following points reflect what we would consider to be the ideal experience for us and whilst we are aware that it may not be possible to fulfil some of these wishes, we would like to maintain a flexible approach all round with full consultation at all stages in order to have a positive experience.

VAGINAL BREECH DELIVERY — 1ST STAGE OF LABOUR

1. I would like to start labour spontaneously and not be induced unless it is decided that the baby might be at risk.
2. I would like an active 1st stage of labour, at home with my midwife (my sister) monitoring the fetal heart regularly with her pocket sonic-aid. Unless there are reasons to transfer early, I would like to stay at home until labour is well established, the cervix being well dilated (but obviously not leaving it too late).
3. Once in hospital I would like my labour support to be continued by Philip (my husband), Penny (my sister and independent midwife) and Sue (an independent midwife who has been sharing my antenatal care with Penny).
4. I would prefer intermittent to continual fetal monitoring without a fetal scalp electrode (unless there was suspected fetal distress), and I would prefer telemetry

in order to enable me to move around to encourage normal physiological processes, help with pain, etc.

5. No acceleration with oxytocics unless necessary.

6. *Epidural?* I would prefer not to have one if I'm coping well but recognize that if I'm not relaxed for delivery it would be a useful aid.

2ND STAGE AND DELIVERY

1. Any chance of not being in lithotomy? I really would prefer to be upright on the birthing bed in a suitable position.

2. *Episiotomy?* I'd prefer *not* and if it is considered completely necessary would rather have a mid-line cut.

3. *Forceps?* Any chance of delivering the head without forceps – Mauriceau–Smellie–Veit method?

3RD STAGE

1. No syntometrine unless necessary.

2. Unless the baby needs resuscitation I would prefer the cord not to be cut until the placenta is delivered by me, in an upright position, baby at the breast.

3. I don't mind the baby having Vitamin K orally.

CAESAREAN DELIVERY

1. Under epidural if possible.

2. Philip and Penny present in supporting role.

3. Baby to breast straight away if well.

4. If general anaesthetic could Penny be there as an observer in order to fill me in on the experience afterwards?

5. If an elective Caesarean section would it be possible for me to start labour normally and then have the section in early labour?

POSTNATALLY

1. I would like to go home as soon as possible since my sister (midwife) will be staying with me full time to follow through my postnatal care.

2. I would like the baby next to me, or in bed with me, all the time.

3. I want to fully breastfeed on demand – please no water or dextrose.

Thank you.

Julie says that when thinking ahead to the birth she was 'very scared . . . it was like a bad dream'. But she was relieved when a scan at 38 weeks revealed that her pelvis was large enough for her to deliver the baby vaginally. She felt grateful that she was at a hospital where breech babies were not delivered by Caesarean as a matter of course.

This is what happened when she went into labour:

Labour first stage

Saturday/Sunday Minor contractions, heavy shows. Feeling relieved now that Penny has arrived from London and is with me.

Sunday 7 p.m. Contractions increasing. Labour really starts. Eat a large pasta meal and make sure everything is packed for hospital. Need Philip near me now at all times.

9 p.m. Waters break. Ring up hospital who want us to come in immediately.

10 p.m. Penny drives Philip and me to hospital where we meet midwife, Kathy. From the first moment I meet her, she makes me feel very positive about being in hospital. I give Kathy the birth plan. She is wonderful and makes me feel anything is possible, encouragingly shows us the birthing bed, rocking chair. Contractions are now very strong and painful, needing my full concentration. With each contraction I need to hold on to Philip.

10.15 p.m. Joanna, a midwife who is also a homeopath, whose childbirth classes we attended, arrives.

10.30 p.m. Meet Dr Livingstone, the registrar. Together we go through the birth plan. His reaction is very positive – what a relief! At this point he cannot commit himself, but is happy about delivering the baby on the end of the bed, trying without drugs for pain relief and avoiding forceps. He basically says, 'Let's see how it goes.' His approach and attitude make all the difference in the world. Dr Livingstone goes to bed leaving Kathy, Joanna, Philip, Penny and me to finish first stage.

Monday 11 p.m. to 6 a.m. To the background of music (mostly Mozart), supported by Philip, Penny and Joanna, I go through the first stage, changing position from the rocking chair to sitting on the bed. The fetal heart and contraction monitors are taken off, except for occasional readings between 1 and 5 a.m. When it is in use Kathy's hand holds it – really good of her, as I find the straps uncomfortable. In between contractions I suck ice cold water from a sponge and the occasional glucose tablet. Joanna gives me homeopathic remedies. I try not to look at the clock as I find this stage endless.

At the height of every contraction my friends give help by close eye contact. I remember vividly Penny and Joanna's strong and compassionate eyes saying, 'You can do it,' 'You're doing brilliantly.' And thinking, 'I'm not, and want pain relief.'

I ask in desperation, 'How much longer, how many more hours?' Their reply is honest, but not comforting, yet I am glad of their honesty as I continue to trust them. At peaks of contractions Penny holds my head and I feel anchored and able to cope.

I feel complete dependency on Philip, Penny and Joanna – need all their strength, think if Philip breaks down now that will be it – he doesn't. His strength is solid. I want to cry but know I have to keep strong.

As I am having no drugs for pain relief my body's own pain defences come into action – I hallucinate and feel completely out of my head. I watch a cupboard on the wall in front of me become larger and smaller over and over again.

6 a.m. Transition comes. It feels like the end of the world – I've had enough – no break from the intense pain. At this point Kathy comes in, does an internal and says I am fully dilated. Penny and Joanna jump up and down with delight. I hold on to Philip who continues to give me unfailing strength.

Labour second stage

Monday 6 to 7.20 a.m. I now want to stand up. When I feel a contraction I link my hands around Philip's neck and, still standing, push as this overriding urge comes.

6.30 a.m. Dr Livingstone arrives and to everyone's surprise decides to take on the delivery as he finds us – standing. The lights are still dimmed, as they have been throughout. He lies down on the floor, between my legs.

This is the stage I have most dreaded and always imagined I would not be able to cope with. To my surprise it is not painful, but an indescribable, overpowering, opening sensation that makes me want to shout each time I push.

I continue with my hands around Philip's neck and let him take all my weight as I push down.

Penny kneels on the floor next to Dr Livingstone and tells me what is happening in an encouraging and reassuring way. 'Baby's leg is just coming out now.' Although Dr Livingstone offers to tell us the baby's sex, and for me to hold the baby's legs as they are coming out, I refuse, as I just want to concentrate on pushing and getting our baby born. Still I cannot believe or take for granted that our baby will be all right.

It is amazing to see my baby's legs hanging from inside me. I remember thinking, 'I've been pregnant for the last nine months and now I can see there really *is* a baby inside me!' Dr Livingstone, with his hands, gently delivers our baby – NO FORCEPS, NO EPISIOTOMY.

7.20 a.m. Our baby girl is born, followed straight away by the placenta landing on Dr Livingstone's head! (He is still lying on the floor.) The baby is rushed away by the surprised and slightly anxious paediatrician, but everything is fine. I have a beautiful healthy daughter. Dr Livingstone seems as delighted as us.

I walk over to see her as she lies on the paediatrician's 'table', eyes wide open, calmly and alertly taking everything in. She is so beautiful!

I have feelings of such love for Philip, Penny, Joanna, Kathy and Dr Livingstone – and overwhelming love for Amy, who is so precious as not to be real. In fact, at first I do not want to hold her – I am shaky, so am glad for Philip to cuddle her. I feel proud that I have not taken any drugs for pain relief. It is wonderful to have her suckling straight away from my breast. I feel so grateful to everyone! As the moments go by I realize more and more just what Dr Livingstone's bold and skilful actions have enabled me and my baby to experience. I shall always be grateful to him.

Because I had no drugs for pain relief and a positive and straightforward birth I can leave hospital after only five hours and go home where Penny will continue my postnatal care for ten days.

However straightforward your pregnancy, and even if you very much want an autonomous birth, it is wise to consider the possibility of Caesarean section and what a Caesarean birth plan would be like. One woman in every nine in Britain and one in four in the USA ends up with Caesarean birth. Some women do not want to consider the possibility because they believe that if they do so it will act as a kind of 'softening up' process and make them more ready to think that a section is really necessary. On the other hand, a woman who has not thought ahead to what she would want if a Caesarean seemed the safest manner of delivery tends to be thrown off course, unable to act assertively and make any decisions herself. Here is one woman's Caesarean birth plan. Your own may be very different, but the issues with which she deals are all ones which you may want to consider.

CAESAREAN BIRTH PLAN REQUESTS

I should like to
  wait for labour to start before the Caesarean section is performed;
  discuss all procedures in advance;
  have my partner with me during prepping, administration of anaesthesia and
    the birth;
  be shaved only as necessary;
  be given medication only after receiving information about it;
  have epidural anaesthesia for the operation;
  if I should need general anaesthesia, have my partner stay with me so that he
    can hold the baby immediately after delivery;
  have no curtain obstructing my view;
  have a mirror so that I can watch the birth if I wish;
  hold the baby immediately after delivery and breastfeed on the delivery table;
  have baby stay with me all the time unless he/she needs to be taken to the
    nursery;
  be consulted about it first if I am awake and baby needs to be taken to the
    nursery;
  have my partner and the baby go with me to the recovery room;
  know that no artificial milk will be given to the baby;
  breastfeed on demand;
  not be separated from the baby unless I wish it;
  have a visit from my 3-year-old, and a chance for her to meet the baby, as soon
    as possible.

If a baby needs to go to the special care nursery, you can also make
contingency plans. You may, for example, sketch out something like this:

If our baby has to be in the nursery we would welcome the opportunity of un-
    restricted visiting.
We should like to be able to touch, and if possible hold, our baby.
It would help a great deal if all procedures and any medication given to the baby
    could be explained to us.
Since I plan to breastfeed my baby if possible, I want to use a breast pump and
    should like to know that my baby will not, unless absolutely necessary, have
    any artificial feeds.
We should like to be kept fully informed about our baby's condition at all times.
If our baby is severely ill and there is no hope, we wish to have all tubes and other
    apparatus removed so that the baby can die in our arms.
If our baby has a severe handicap we should like full discussion with the paedia-
    trician before any drug treatment is started or surgery embarked on, to con-
    sider whether it would be better for the child to have nurturing only, and
    explore all options.

You may feel that it demands too much of you to contemplate the death of a baby. Some women believe that if they let themselves acknowledge that there is even the faintest possibility of such a thing happening this can somehow make it more likely to occur in reality. It is understandable that we don't want to dwell on such thoughts. Yet many of us secretly fear that we may lose the baby and the dread is made still worse by feeling isolated and alone with it. It can seem 'bad taste' to voice such fears, largely because it tends to disturb other people's equanimity and make them anxious – especially care-givers. The result is that when things go terribly wrong and a baby dies – and even when there is the highest level of care it must be remembered that four out of every 1,000 babies die at or around the time of birth – a woman is completely unprepared emotionally and actions are undertaken on her behalf which are very different from those she would have wanted herself.

Even if you do not think in terms of a 'plan', this is a subject which it can be helpful to discuss with your partner or someone else close to you so that, to a certain extent at least, you can sort out in your own mind how you would wish things to be and the degree to which you would want to be involved in making decisions about what happens. Here are one woman's thoughts about this. She did not hand this to her doctor, but had it in her suitcase packed for hospital, in case it was needed:

> In the rare event that my baby dies at birth I should wish
> to see and hold the baby;
> to have undisturbed time alone with the baby;
> not to be on a ward or corridor with mothers of new-borns;
> to have a private room, with a bed for my partner too;
> not to have tranquillizers or drugs which blunt or delay grieving;
> to arrange a funeral ourselves.

Thinking about such choices, making painful decisions, looking at the whole birth experience with openness and honesty – all this helps to forge self-confidence and prepare you to be an active birth-giver instead of a passive patient, and – more than that – to be in touch with the heart of life and to grow in new awareness and understanding of yourself and others.

AFTERWORD

Throughout this book I have been exploring choices and decision-making. As you will have realized, that is not a simple matter of stating preferences as if you were selecting dishes from a menu. If your care-givers are so accommodating that it seems as if that is all that is involved, it is worth thinking about who composed the menu in the first place, since it may be that you are being offered a very limited range of choices. When hospitals institute their own birth plans there is danger that this both formalizes and restricts a woman's choice so that consideration of matters which do not appear on the birth plan can be quietly and politely discouraged, and in the face of such an apparently liberal attitude on the part of the hospital it seems demanding to explore and discuss other issues.

Knowledge brings power. But the profession of medicine restricts access to knowledge for all those who are not within its membership. Whereas at first it seems that choosing how you want to have your baby is a matter of learning about pregnancy and birth and making decisions based on that information, it soon becomes obvious that the information we need is closely guarded. This is especially clear when we enquire what goes on inside hospitals. We are fed crumbs of information which those controlling the institution allow us to receive, and even that is often inaccurate.

Getting information entails acquiring power. It is a political act. It means joining together with others who have similar concerns to work for social change.

Through striving to achieve autonomy in childbirth – the biological act which epitomizes woman's role as mother, nurturer and homemaker – conformists become non-conformists, assimilators become dissidents, charming, polite, compliant women become political activists.

Birth is not only a matter of producing a top-quality baby, a first-class product, as many obstetricians believe. Nor is it only a matter of the mother's physical well-being or even her emotional fulfilment. The way we experience pregnancy and birth today raises political issues which have profound significance for our own lives, for those of our children and for all those who come after us.

REFERENCES

Chapter 1: Curtain up on Pregnancy

1. Barbara Katz Rothman, *The Tentative Pregnancy: Prenatal Diagnosis and the Future of Motherhood* (Viking, New York, 1986).

Chapter 2: The Early Weeks

1. Barbara Pickard, 'Vitamin B6 during pregnancy', *Nutrition and Health*, 1 (1982), 78–84.
2. F. E. Hilton and R. Leitch, *The Physiology of Human Pregnancy*, 2nd edn (Blackwell, Oxford, 1971).
3. K. Niswander and M. Gordon, *The Collaborative Perinatal Study: The Women and Their Pregnancies* (W. B. Saunders, Philadelphia, 1972).
4. 'Vaginal bleeding in early pregnancy' (editorial), *British Medical Journal*, 6 (1980), 470.

Chapter 3: Drugs and Health

1. *The Health Consequences of Smoking for Women: A Report of the Surgeon General* (US Department of Health, Education and Welfare, Washington DC, 1980).
2. K. Praeger *et al.*, 'Smoking and drinking behavior before and during pregnancy of married mothers of live-born infants and still-born infants', *Public Health Reports*, 99 (1984), 117–23.
3. N. R. Butler and E. D. Alberman (eds.), *Perinatal Problems: The Second Report of the 1958 British Perinatal Mortality Survey* (Churchill Livingstone, Edinburgh, 1969).
4. M. Stjernfeldt *et al.*, 'Maternal smoking during pregnancy and risk of childhood cancer', *Lancet*, 1 (1986), 1350–52.
5. N. R. Butler and H. Goldstein, 'Smoking in pregnancy and subsequent child development', *British Medical Journal*, 4 (1973), 573–5.
6. Peter C. Buchan, 'Cigarette smoking in pregnancy and fetal hyperviscosity', *British Medical Journal*, 286 (1983), 13–15.
7. M. B. Meyer and J. A. Tunascia, 'Maternal smoking, pregnancy complications and perinatal mortality', *American Journal of Obstetrics and Gynecology*, 128 (1977), 494.
8. D. O. Ho-Yen *et al.*, 'Why smoke fewer cigarettes?', *British Medical Journal*, 284 (1982), 1905–7.
9. R. Olegard *et al.*, 'Effects on the child of alcohol abuse during pregnancy', *Acta Paediatrica Scandinavica*, 275, supplement (Sweden, 1979), 112–21.
10. J. W. Hanson *et al.*, 'Effects of moderate alcohol consumption during pregnancy on fetal growth and morphogenesis', *Journal of Paediatrics*, 92 : 3 (1978), 457–60.

11. R. J. Sokol et al., 'Alcohol abuse during pregnancy: an epidemiologic study', Alcoholism Clinics in Experimental Research, 4:2 (1980), 135–45.
12. J. Kline et al., 'Drinking during pregnancy and spontaneous abortion', Lancet, 2 (1980), 176–80.
13. S. Harlap and P. H. Shiono, 'Alcohol, smoking and incidence of spontaneous abortion in the first and second trimesters', Lancet, 2 (1980), 173–6.
14. H. O. Rosett et al., 'Patterns of alcohol consumption and fetal development', Obstetrics and Gynecology, 61:5 (1983), 539–46.
15. P. L. Doering and R. B. Stewart, 'The extent and character of drug consumption during pregnancy', Journal of the American Medical Association, 239 (1978), 843–6.
16. Yvonne Brackbill et al., Medication in Maternity (University of Michigan Press, Ann Arbor, 1985).
17. ibid.
18. Bruce H. Wooley, 'Herbal pharmacology and toxicology', Journal of Collegium Aesculatium (December 1983), 1–11.
19. R. K. Siegel, 'Ginseng abuse syndrome – problems with the panacea', Journal of the American Medical Association, 241 (1979), 1614–15.

Chapter 4: Choosing the Right Food

1. Madeleine H. Shearer, 'Malnutrition in middle-class pregnant women', Birth and the Family Journal, 7:1 (Spring 1980), 27–35.
2. A. Stewart Truswell, 'Nutrition for pregnancy', British Medical Journal, 291 (1985), 263–6.
3. John Dobbing (ed.), Prevention of Spina Bifida and Other Neural Tube Defects (Academic Press, London, 1983).
4. K. Laurence et al., 'Increased risk of recurrence of pregnancies complicated by fatal neural tube defects in mothers receiving poor diets and possible benefit of dietary counselling', British Medical Journal, 281 (1980), 1592–4.
5. R. C. Goodlin et al., 'Clinical signs of normal plasma volume expansion during pregnancy', American Journal of Obstetrics and Gynecology, 145 (1983), 1001–9.
6. Thomas H. Brewer, Metabolic Toxaemia of Late Pregnancy (Keats Publishing Inc. [27 Pine Street, New Canaan, Connecticut 06840], 1982).
7. R. Collins et al., 'Overview of randomised trials of diuretics in pregnancy', British Medical Journal, 290 (1985), 17–23.
8. A. Lechtig et al., 'Effect of food supplementation during pregnancy on birthweight', Pediatrics, 56 (1975), 508–19. D. Rush et al., 'A randomised controlled trial of pre-natal nutritional supplementation in New York', Pediatrics, 65 (1980), 685–97.
9. O. A. C. Viegas et al., 'Dietary protein energy supplementation of pregnant Asian mothers at Sorrento, Birmingham, I: Unselective during second and third trimesters', British Medical Journal, 285 (1982), 589–91.
10. O. A. C. Viegas et al., 'Dietary protein energy supplementation of pregnant Asian mothers at Sorrento, Birmingham, II: Selective during third trimester only', British Medical Journal, 285 (1982), 592–5.

Chapter 5: Exercise

1. Susan L. Woodward, 'How does strenuous maternal exercise affect the fetus? A review', *Birth*, 8:1 (1981), 17–23.
2. J. F. Newhall, 'Scubadiving in pregnancy', *American Journal of Obstetrics and Gynecology*, 140 (1981), 893–4.
3. G. Turner and I. Unsworth, 'Intrauterine bends?', *Lancet*, 1 (1982), 905.
4. M. E. Bolton, 'Scubadiving and fetal well-being', *Undersea Biomedical Research*, 7 (1980), 183–9.
5. Frederick Leboyer, *Inner Beauty Inner Light: Yoga for Pregnant Women* (Borzoi Books, New York, 1978).
6. C. A. Collins *et al.*, 'Maternal and fetal responses to a maternal aerobic exercise program', *American Journal of Obstetrics and Gynecology*, 145 (1983), 702.
7. Janet Balaskas: *Active Birth* (Unwin, London, 1983); *The Active Birth Partners' Handbook* (Sidgwick & Jackson, London, 1984).
8. Sheila Kitzinger, *Women as Mothers* (Vintage Books, New York, 1980). R. J. Atwood, 'Parturitional posture and related birth behaviour', *Acta Obstetrica et Ginecologica Scandinavica*, 57, supplement (Sweden, 1976), 1–25. R. W. Wertz and D. C. Wertz, *Lying In: A History of Childbirth in America* (Free Press, New York, 1977). G. Engelmann, *Labour among Primitive People* (St Louis, 1882).
9. P. Dunn, 'Obstetrics delivery today, for better or worse?', *Lancet*, 1 (1976), 790–93. W. I. Hampton, 'Practical considerations for the routine application of left lateral Sims' position for vaginal delivery', *American Journal of Obstetrics and Gynecology*, 131 (1978), 129–33. M. A. Hugo, 'A look at maternal positions during labour', *Nurse Midwifery*, XXII (1977), 26–7. Y. C. Lieu, 'Effects of an upright position during labour', *American Journal of Nursing*, 74 (1974), 2203–5. C. Mendez-Bauer *et al.*, 'Effects of standing position on spontaneous uterine contractility and other aspects of labor', *Journal of Perinatal Medicine*, 3 (1975), 89–100. I. N. Mitre, 'The Influence of maternal position on duration of the active phase of labor', *International Journal of Gynaecology and Obstetrics*, 12 (1974), 181–3.
10. A. M. Flynn and J. Kelly, 'Continuous fetal monitoring in the ambulant patient in labour', *British Medical Journal*, 2 (1976), 842–3.

Chapter 6: The Environment in Pregnancy

1. W. R. Lee, 'Working with visual display units', *British Medical Journal*, 291 (1985), 989–91.
2. A. Kurpa *et al.*, 'Birth defects and video display terminals', *Lancet*, 2 (1984), 1339.
3. V. J. Bayne, 'A trade union response to the allegations of reproductive hazards from VDUs', in B. G. Pearce (ed.), *Allegations of Reproductive Hazards from VDUs* (Humane Technology, Loughborough, Leics., 1984), 161–75.
4. L. D. Longo, 'Environmental pollution and pregnancy: risks and uncertainties for the fetus and the infant', *American Journal of Obstetrics and Gynecology*, 137 (1980), 162–73.
5. L. D. Longo, 'The biological effects of carbon monoxide on the pregnant woman, fetus and newborn infant', *American Journal of Obstetrics and Gynecology*, 129 (1977), 69.

6. Sheila McKechnie, 'Reproductive hazards in employment: protect the fetus, yes, but not at the expense of the adult woman', *Medical World* (4 June 1981), 5.
7. K. Hemminki *et al.*, 'Spontaneous abortions in hospital staff engaged in sterilising instruments with chemical agents', *British Medical Journal*, 285 (1982), 1461–3.

Chapter 7: Emotional Changes

1. R. Kumar and K. Robson, 'Previous induced abortion and antenatal depression in primipara', *Psychology and Medicine*, 8 (1978), 711–15.
2. Richard L. Naeye and Ellen C. Peters, 'Causes and consequences of premature rupture of fetal membranes', *Lancet*, 1 (1980), 192–4.

Chapter 8: What Kind of Prenatal Care?

1. Jean Donnison, *Midwives and Medical Men* (Heinemann Educational, London, 1977). Margot Edwards and Mary Waldorf, *Reclaiming Birth* (The Crossing Press, New York, 1984): chapter on 'The midwife question'. Margarita Artschwager Kay, *Anthropology of Human Birth* (F. A. Davis Company, Philadelphia, 1982). Shelly Romalis (ed.), *Childbirth Alternatives to Medical Control* (University of Texas Press, 1981). Richard W. Wertz and Dorothy C. Wertz, *Lying In: A History of Childbirth in America* (The Free Press, New York, 1977).
2. Shirley Ardener (ed.), *Defining Females* (Croom Helm, London, 1978). Sheila Kitzinger, *Women as Mothers* (Fontana, London, 1978). Carol P. MacCormack (ed.), *Ethnography of Fertility and Birth* (Academic Press, London, 1982).
3. Sheila Kitzinger, op. cit. Sheila Kitzinger, 'The social context of birth: some comparisons between childbirth in Jamaica and Britain', in Carol P. MacCormack (ed.), op. cit.
4. Wendy D. Savage, 'Antenatal care in Britain', *Nursing*, 21 (1980), 909–11.
5. See Alison Macfarlane and Miranda Mugford, *Birth Counts: Statistics of Pregnancy and Childbirth* (HMSO, London, 1984).
6. *Infant and Perinatal Mortality 1980* (Office of Population Censuses and Surveys, London, 1982).
7. As reported in the *Guardian*, 13 September 1984.
8. Ann Oakley, *The Captured Womb: A History of the Medical Care of Pregnant Women* (Blackwell, Oxford, 1984).
9. ibid.
10. Marion H. Hall *et al.*, 'Is routine antenatal care worth while?', *Lancet*, 2 (1980), 78–80.
11. ibid.
12. Mary J. Houston and Lesley Page, *Midwifery: Practice and Research* (Churchill Livingstone, Edinburgh, forthcoming).
13. Gordon Bourne, *Pregnancy* (Pan, London, 1975).
14. Ann Oakley, *Women Confined: Towards a Sociology of Childbirth* (Martin Robertson, Oxford, 1980). Hilary Graham, 'Problems in antenatal care' (paper presented at DHSS/Child Poverty Action Group Conference, 1978). Sally Macintyre, 'Consumer reaction to present-day antenatal services', in

Luke Zander and Geoffrey Chamberlain (eds.), *Pregnancy Care for the 1980s* (Royal Society of Medicine and Macmillan, 1984). Sheila Kitzinger, 'What do women want?', in John Studd (ed.), *The Management of Labour* (Blackwell Scientific Publications, Oxford, 1985).

15. Sarah Robinson, 'Responsibilities of midwives and medical staff: findings from the National Survey', *Midwives Chronicle*, March 1985.
16. G. Chamberlain, *et al.*, (*British Births*, Heinemann, London, 1970).
17. ibid.
18. H. D. Kleinert *et al.*, 'What is the value of home blood pressure measurement in patients with mild hypertension?', *Hypertension*, 6 (1984), 574–8.
19. E. Brien *et al.*, 'Blood pressure measurement: current practice and future trends', *British Medical Journal*, 290 (1985), 729–34.
20. R. M. Carey *et al.*, 'The Charlottesville blood pressure survey: value of repeated blood pressure measurements', *Journal of the American Medical Association*, 236 (1972), 847–51.
21. Rory Collins *et al.*, 'Overview of randomised trials of diuretics in pregnancy', *British Medical Journal*, 290 (1985), 17–23.
22. J. Fidler *et al.*, 'Randomised controlled comparative study of methyldopa and oxprenolol in treatment of hypertension in pregnancy', *British Medical Journal*, 286 (1983), 1927–30.
23. M. Ounstead and C. W. G. Redman, letter, *British Medical Journal*, 290 (1985), 1080.
24. Collins *et al.*, op. cit.

Chapter 9: Deciding about Special Tests

1. J. Murphy *et al.*, 'Conservative management of pregnancy in diabetic women', *British Medical Journal*, 288 (1984), 1203.
2. 'Second report of UK Collaborative Study on A F P in Relation to Neural Tube Defects', *Lancet*, 2 (1979), 651–62.
3. J. B. Holton, 'Assessment of fetal immaturity and prediction of respiratory distress syndrome', in A. C. Turnbull and F. P. Woodward (eds.), *Prevention of Handicap through Antenatal Care* (Elsevier, Amsterdam, 1976).
4. B. N. Hibbard *et al.*, 'Can we afford screening for neural tube defects? The South Wales experience', *British Medical Journal*, 290 (1985), 293–5.
5. Professor John Edwards, personal communication.
6. Medical Research Council Working Party on Amniocentesis, 'An assessment of the hazards of amniocentesis', *British Journal of Obstetrics and Gynaecology*, 85, Supplement 2 (1978).
7. L. N. Reece, 'The estimation of fetal maturity by a new method of X-ray cephalometry: its bearing on clinical midwifery', *Proceedings of the Royal Society of Medicine* (18 January 1935), 489–504; quoted in Ann Oakley, *The Captured Womb: A History of the Medical Care of Pregnant Women* (Blackwell, Oxford, 1984).
8. R. W. A. Salmond, 'The uses and value of radiology in obstetrics', in F. J. Browne (ed.), *Antenatal and Postnatal Care* (Churchill, London, 1935); quoted in Ann Oakley, op. cit.
9. Ann Oakley, op. cit.

10. A. Stewart *et al.*, 'Malignant disease in childhood and diagnostic irradiation in utero', *Lancet*, 2 (1956), 447.

11. Doris Haire, 'Fetal effects of ultrasound: a growing controversy', *Journal of Nurse Midwifery*, 29:4 (1984).

12. H. F. Stewart and M. E. Stratmeyer, *An Overview of Ultrasound: Theory, Measurement, Medical Applications and Biological Effects*, HHS Publication FDA 82–8190 (Bureau of Radiological Health, Food and Drug Administration, 1982).

13. American College of Obstetricians and Gynecologists, *Diagnostic Ultrasound in Obstetrics and Gynecology*, ACOG Technical Bulletin No. 63 (1981). Office of Technology Assessment, 'Policy implications of the computed tomography (CT) scanner: an update', in *Research and Development of CT and other Diagnostic Imaging Technologies* (Washington DC, 1981).

14. M. Edwards and P. Simkin, *Obstetric Tests and Technology: A Consumer's Guide* (The Pennypress, Seattle, 1980).

15. American College of Obstetricians and Gynecologists, op. cit.

16. J. P. Neilson, S. P. Munjanja and C. R. Whitfield, 'Screening for small-for-dates fetuses: a controlled trial', *British Medical Journal*, 289 (1984), 1170–82.

17. B. Bolsen, 'Question of risk still hovers over routine prenatal use of ultrasound', *Journal of the American Medical Association*, 247 (1982), 2195–7. H. F. Stewart and M. E. Stratmeyer, op. cit.

18. D. Liebeskind *et al.*, 'Diagnostic ultrasound: effects on DNA and growth patterns of animal cells', *Radiology*, 131:1 (1979), 177–84.

19. American College of Obstetricians and Gynecologists, op. cit.

20. Penny Simkin *et al.*, *Pregnancy, Childbirth and the Newborn* (Meadowbrook Press, Deephaven, Minnesota, 1984). International Childbirth Education Association, *Diagnostic Ultrasound in Obstetrics* (1983).

21. National Institutes of Health, *Antenatal Diagnosis*, NIH Publication No. 79 (US Department of Health, Education and Welfare, 1973).

22. R. E. Myers, 'Maternal anxiety and fetal death', in L. Zichella and P. Pancheri (eds.), *Psychoendocrinology in Reproduction* (Elsevier, Amsterdam, 1979).

23. A. Grant and P. Mohide, 'Screening and diagnostic tests in antenatal care', in M. Enkin and I. Chalmers (eds.), *Effectiveness and Satisfaction in Antenatal Care* (Spastics International, London, 1982).

24. Richard Hamilton, *The Herpes Book* (Houghton Mifflin, Boston, 1980).

25. Zane A. Brown, 'Herpes update' (paper presented at Utah Perinatal Conference, Salt Lake City, October 1985).

26. J. F. Pearson and J. B. Weaver, 'Fetal activity and fetal wellbeing: an evaluation', *British Medical Journal*, 1 (1976), 1305–7.

27. R. Homburg *et al.*, 'Management of patients with a live fetus and cessation of fetal movement', *British Journal of Obstetrics and Gynaecology*, 87 (1980), 804–7.

Chapter 10: Saying What You Want

1. Helen Roberts, *Patient Patients* (Pandora Press, London, 1985).

2. Ann Oakley, *Women Confined: Towards a Society of Childbirth* (Martin Robertson, Oxford, 1980).

Chapter 11: Birth Plans

1. Harold Francis, 'Obstetrics: a consumer oriented service? The case against', *Maternal and Child Health*, 10:3 (1985), 69–72.
2. R. P. Lederman *et al.*, 'The relationship of maternal anxiety, plasma catecholamines and plasma cortisol to progress in labour', *American Journal of Obstetrics and Gynecology*, 132 (1973), 495.
3. Michael Klein, 'Contracting for trust in family practice obstetrics', *Canadian Family Physician*, 29 (1983), 2225–7.
4. R. Sosa *et al.*, 'The effect of support on perinatal problems', *New England Journal of Medicine*, 303 (1980), 597–600.
5. Sheila Kitzinger, *Women as Mothers* (Fontana, London, 1978).
6. S. V. D. Anderson, 'Siblings at birth', *Birth*, 6 (1979), 80–87.
7. R. Campbell *et al.*, 'Perinatal mortality and place of delivery', *Population Trends*, 20 (1982), 9–12.
8. R. Campbell, 'Statistics and policy making in the maternity services' (lecture in symposium, Royal Society of Medicine, December 1984).
9. Iain Chalmers, National Perinatal Epidemiology Unit, Oxford (personal communication).
10. Marjorie Tew, 'The case against hospital deliveries: the statistical evidence', in Sheila Kitzinger and John A. Davies (eds.), *The Place of Birth* (Oxford University Press, 1978). Marjorie Tew, 'Is home a safer place?', *Health and Social Service Journal* (12 September 1980), 702–5.
11. J. F. Murphy *et al.*, 'Planned and unplanned deliveries at home: implications of a changing ratio', *British Medical Journal*, 298 (1984), 1429–32.
12. S. M. I. Damstra-Wijmenga, 'Home confinement: the positive results in Holland', *Journal of the Royal College of Practitioners*, 34 (1984), 425–30.
13. G. W. Taylor *et al.*, 'How safe is general practitioner obstetrics?', *Lancet*, 2 (1980), 1287–9.
14. Michael Klein *et al.*, 'A comparison of low risk women booked for delivery in two different systems of care', *British Journal of Obstetrics and Gynaecology*, 90 (1983), 118–22 and 123–8. Michael Klein *et al.*, 'Booking for maternity care: a comparison of two systems', Occasional Paper 31 (Royal College of General Practitioners, 1985).
15. R. C. Goodlin and I. B. Frederick, 'Postpartum vulvar edema associated with the birthing chair', *American Journal of Obstetrics and Gynecology*, 146:3 (1984), 334.

Chapter 12: Getting in Touch with Your Baby

1. D. Purpura, 'Consciousness', *Behavior Today* (2 June 1975), 494.
2. C. M. Nistretta and R. M. Bradley, 'Taste in utero: theoretical considerations', in J. M. Weiffenbach (ed.), *Taste and Development: the Genesis of Sweet Preference* (US Printing Office, Washington DC, 1977), 51–69.
3. K. C. Pratt *et al.*, *The Behavior of the Newborn Infant* (Ohio State University Press, Columbus, 1930).
4. K. R. Kobre and L. R. Lipsitt, 'A negative contrast effect in newborns', *Journal of Experimental Child Psychology*, 14 (1972), 81–91.

5. C. K. Crook, 'Taste perception in the newborn infant', *Infant Behaviour and Development*, 1 (1978), 52–69.
6. R. Artal *et al.*, 'Fetal response to sound', *Contemporary Ob/Gyn*, 5 (1975).
7. M. Clements, 'Observations on certain aspects of neonatal behaviour in response to auditory stimuli' (paper presented at the 5th International Congress of Psychosomatic Obstetrics and Gynaecology, Rome, 1977).
8. R. G. Eisenberg, 'Auditory behaviors in the human neonate', *Journal of Auditory Research*, 5 (1965), 159–77.
9. D. B. Chamberlain, *Consciousness at Birth: A Review of the Empirical Evidence* (Chamberlain Communications, San Diego, 1983), 26–49.
10. W. S. Condon and L. W. Sander, 'Neonate movement is synchronised with adult speech: interaction or participation and language acquisition', *Science*, 183 (1974), 99–101.
11. N. Hack and M. Klaus, *The Amazing Newborn* (film distributed by Ross Laboratories, Columbus, Ohio, 1976).
12. A. DeCasper and W. Fifer, 'Of human bonding: newborns prefer their mother's voices', *Science*, 208 (1980), 1174–6.
13. H. Truby and J. Lind, 'Cry sounds of the newborn infant', in J. Lind (ed.), *Newborn Infant Cry* (*Acta Paediatrica Scandinavica*, 163, supplement, Sweden, 1965), 7–59.
14. M. Wertheimer, 'Psychomotor coordination of auditory and visual space at birth', *Science*, 134 (1961), 1692.
15. L. Salk, 'The role of the heart beat in the relations between mother and infant', *Scientific American* (May 1973), 24–9.
16. H. P. Roffwarg *et al.*, 'Ontogenetic development of the human sleep–dream cycle', *Science*, 152 (1966), 604–19.
17. A. B. Roberts *et al.*, 'Fetal activity in 100 normal third trimester pregnancies', *British Journal of Obstetrics and Gynaecology*, 87 (1980), 480–84.
18. Chamberlain, op. cit. E. E. Van Woerden Petal, 'Distribution of movements within behavioural states of the human fetus' (paper presented at the European Congress of Perinatal Medicine, Dublin, 1984). J. I. P. de Vries, 'Incidence of specific movement patterns during the first half of gestation' (paper presented at the European Congress of Perinatal Medicine, Dublin, 1984). K. Maeda *et al.*, 'New ultrasonic Doppler fetal actogram and the analysis of FHR changes related to fetal movement' (paper presented at the European Congress of Perinatal Medicine, Dublin, 1984).
19. Chamberlain, op cit.
20. J. F. Pearson and J. B. Weaver, 'Fetal activity and fetal wellbeing: an evaluation', *British Medical Journal*, 1 (1976), 1305–7.

Chapter 13: On the Threshold of the Unknown

1. Clare M. Andrews, 'Changing fetal position', *Journal of Nurse Midwifery*, 25: 1 (1980), 7–12.
2. G. R. Evaldson *et al.*, 'Premature rupture of the membranes and ascending infection', *British Journal of Obstetrics and Gynaecology*, 89 (1982), 793.
3. P. Duff *et al.*, 'Management of premature rupture of membranes on unfavorable cervix in term pregnancy', *Obstetrics and Gynecology*, 63 (1984), 69.

4. M. F. Shutte *et al.*, 'Management of premature rupture of membranes: the risk of vaginal examination to the infant', *American Journal of Obstetrics and Gynecology*, 146 (1983), 395.

Chapter 15: Dealing with Pain

1. John J. Bonica, 'Labour pain', in Patrick D. Wall and Ronald Melzack (eds.), *Textbook of Pain* (Churchill Livingstone, Edinburgh, 1984).
2. Reported in *Irish Medical Times* (30 March 1984).
3. Grantly Dick-Read, *Childbirth Without Fear*, 9th edn (London, 1942).
4. Bonica, op. cit.
5. Bonica, op. cit.
6. B. M. Morgan *et al.*, 'Epidural analgesia for uneventful labour', *Anaesthesia*, 35 (1980), 57–60.
7. E. Tronick *et al.*, 'Regional obstetric anesthesia and newborn behavior: effect over the first ten days of life', *Pediatrics*, 58 (1976), 94–100.
8. J. F. Pearson and P. Davies, 'The effect of continuous lumbar analgesia on the acid–base status of maternal arterial blood during the first stage of labour', *Journal of Obstetrics and Gynaecology of the British Commonwealth*, 80 (1973), 218–24. J. F. Pearson and P. Davies, 'The effect of continuous lumbar analgesia upon fetal acid–base status during the first stage of labour', *Journal of Obstetrics and Gynaecology of the British Commonwealth* 81 (1974), 971–4.
9. J. W. W. Studd *et al.*, 'The effect of lumbar epidural analgesia on the rate of cervical dilatation and the outcome of labour of spontaneous onset', *British Journal of Obstetrics and Gynaecology*, 87 (1980), 1015–21. J. S. Crawford, 'The second thousand epidural blocks in an obstetric hospital practice', *British Journal of Anaesthetics*, 44 (1972), 1277–96.
10. I. J. Hoult *et al.*, 'Lumbar epidural analgesia in labour: relation to fetal malposition and instrumental delivery', *British Medical Journal*, 1 (1977), 14–16.
11. Crawford, op. cit.
12. Tronick, op. cit.
13. J. W. Scanlon *et al.*, 'Neurobehavioral responses of newborn infants after maternal epidural anesthesia', *Anesthesiology*, 40 (1974), 121–8. Tronick, op. cit. B. A. Liebermann *et al.*, 'The effect of maternally administered pethidine or bupivacaine on fetus and newborn', *British Journal of Obstetrics and Gynaecology*, 86 (1979), 598–806. B. A. Liebermann *et al.*, 'The influence of maternal analgesia on neo-natal behaviour: II, Epidural bupivacaine', *British Journal of Obstetrics and Gynaecology*, 88 (1981), 407–13.
14. Murray W. Enkin, 'Commentary on "Epidural Analgesia" ', *I C E A Review*, 5 (1981), 2.
15. J. J. Bonica, *Obstetric Analgesia and Anaesthesia*, 2nd edn (World Federation of Societies of Anaesthesiologists, Amsterdam, 1980).
16. Michel Odent, *Birth Reborn* (Pantheon, New York, 1984; Fontana, London, 1986).
17. Gayle Peterson, *Birthing Normally: A Personal Growth Approach to Childbirth* (Mind/Body Press, Berkeley, 1981). Claudia Panuthos, *Transformation Through Birth* (Bergin & Garvey, South Hadley, Massachusetts, 1984). Rahima Baldwin and Terra Palmarini, *Pregnant Feelings* (Celestial Arts, Berkeley, 1986).

18. Odent, op. cit.
19. Sheila Kitzinger, *Woman's Experience of Sex* (Penguin, Harmondsworth, 1986). Ina May Gaskin, *Spiritual Midwifery* (The Farm, Summertown, Tennessee, 1978). Odent, op. cit.
20. Ronald Melzack, 'Acupuncture and related forms of folk medicine', in Patrick D. Wall and Ronald Melzack (eds.), *Textbook of Pain* (Churchill Livingstone, Edinburgh, 1984).
21. L. Auginstinsson *et al.*, 'Pain relief during delivery by transcutaneous electrical stimulation', *Pain*, 4 (1977), 59–65.
22. W. S. Kroger, *Clinical and Experimental Hypnosis*, 2nd edn (J. B. Lippincott, Philadelphia, 1977). P. Stone and G. D. Burrows, 'Hypnosis and obstetrics', in G. D. Burrows and L. Dennerstein (eds.), *Handbook of Hypnosis and Psychosomatic Medicine* (Elsevier, Amsterdam, 1980).
23. Jeannine O'Brien Medvin, *Prenatal Yoga and Natural Birth* (Freestone Publishing Company, Monroe, Utah, 1974). Ma Anand Gandha, *Yoga et Maternité* (EPI, Paris, 1979).
24. Barbara A. K. Porter, 'Water and birth: the pros and the cons', editorial in *ICEA News*, 23 (1984), 3.
25. Odent, op. cit.

Chapter 16: Obstetrically Directed Birth

1. Harold Francis, 'Obstetrics: a consumer oriented service? The case against', *Materual and Child Health*, 10:3 (1985), 69.
2. K. O'Driscoll and D. Meagher, *Active Management of Labour* (W. B. Saunders, Eastbourne, 1980).
3. O'Driscoll and Meagher, op. cit.
4. O'Driscoll and Meagher, op. cit.
5. Editorial, *British Journal of Obstetrics and Gynaecology*, 93 (1986), 105–8.
6. James Owen Drife, 'Pre-term rupture of the membrane', *British Medical Journal*, 285 (1982), 583.
7. Sheila Kitzinger: *The Complete Book of Pregnancy and Childbirth* (Knopf, New York, 1980); *Pregnancy and Childbirth* (Penguin, Harmondsworth, 1986).
8. Roberto Caldeyro Barcia, 'Some consequences of obstetrical interference', *Birth and the Family Journal*, 2:2 (1975), 34–7.
9. H. David Banta and Steven B. Thacker, 'Assessing the costs and benefits of electronic fetal monitoring', *Obstetrical and Gynecological Survey*, 38:8, supplement (1979), 627–42.
10. G. Tutera and R. O. Newman, 'Fetal monitoring: its effect on the perinatal mortality and Cesarean section rates and its complications', *American Journal of Obstetrics and Gynecology*, 122 (1975), 750–54.
11. D. M. Okada *et al.*, 'Neonatal scalp abscess and fetal monitoring, factors associated with infection', *American Journal of Obstetrics and Gynecology*, 129 (1977), 185–9.
12. G. S. Sykes *et al.*, 'Fetal distress and the condition of newborn infants', *British Medical Journal*, 287 (1983), 943–8.
13. P. Curzen *et al.*, 'Reliability of cardiotocography in predicting baby's condition at birth', *British Medical Journal*, 289 (1984), 1345–7.

14. Dermot Macdonald et al., 'The Dublin randomised controlled trial of intrapartum electronic fetal heartrate monitoring' (paper presented at 23rd British Congress of Obstetrics and Gynaecology, Birmingham, 1983).

15. R. Schwartz et al., 'Fetal heart rate in labors with intact and with ruptured membranes', Journal of Perinatal Medicine, 1 (1973), 153–65. S. G. Gabbe et al., 'Umbilical cord compression associated with amniotomy', American Journal of Obstetrics and Gynecology, 126 (1976), 353–5. M. Martel et al., 'Blood acid–base at birth in neonates from labors with early and late rupture of membranes', Journal of Pediatrics, 89 (1976), 963–7.

16. Lecturing in refresher course for midwives, Birmingham, 1984.

17. Joseph DeLee, 'The prophylactic forceps question', American Journal of Obstetrics and Gynecology, 1:1 (1920), 34–44.

18. Robert F. Harrison and M. Brennan, 'Fetal outcome after episiotomy or perineal tear' (paper presented at European Congress of Perinatal Medicine, Dublin 1984).

19. Sheila Kitzinger with Rhiannon Walters, Some Women's Experience of Episiotomy, (National Childbirth Trust, London, 1981).

20. Jennifer Sleep et al., 'West Berkshire perineal management trial', British Medical Journal, 289 (1984), 507–90.

21. Sheila Kitzinger and Penny Simkin, Episiotomy and the Second Stage of Labor, 2nd edn (The Pennypress, Seattle, 1986).

22. Cesarean Childbirth, Report of Task Force Office of Research Reporting (National Institutes of Health Consensus Development, Bethesda, Maryland, 1980).

23. Shirley Huchcroft et al., 'Late results of cesarean and vaginal deliveries in cases of breech presentation', Canadian Medical Association Journal, 125 (1982), 726–30.

Chapter 17: Ceremonial Birth Procedures

1. I. E. P. Menzies, The Functioning of Social Systems as a Defence against Anxiety (Pamphlet 3, Tavistock Institute, 1981).

2. Joan Raphael Leff, 'Fears and fantasies of childbirth', Pre and Peri-natal Psychology Association of North America Journal, (Spring 1985), 14–18.

3. H. Kanton et al., 'The value of shaving the pudendal perineal area in delivery preparation', Obstetrics and Gynecology, 25 (1965), 509.

4. Albert E. Long, 'The unshaved perineum at parturition', American Journal of Obstetrics and Gynecology, 99 (1967), 333–6.

5. Mona L. Romney, 'Pre-delivery shaving: an unjustified assault?', Journal of Obstetrics and Gynaecology, 1 (1980), 33–5.

6. 'Preoperative depilation' (editorial), Lancet, 1 (1983), 1311.

7. Mona L. Romney and H. Gordon, 'Is your enema really necessary?', British Medical Journal, 282 (1981), 1268–71.

8. R. Caldeyro-Barcia, 'Physiological and psychological bases for the modern and humanised management of normal labor', Scientific Publication 858 (Latin American Center of Perinatology and Human Development, Montevideo, Uruguay, 1980).

9. T. J. McManus and A. A. Calder, 'Upright posture and the efficiency of labour', *Lancet*, 1 (1978), 72–4.

10. Morag A. Hunter and Delores Williams, 'Mask wearing in the labour ward', *Midwives' Chronicle*, 12 (January 1985), 14.

11. 'Behind the mask' (editorial), *Lancet*, 1 (1981), 197–8.

12. Penny Simkin *et al.*, *Pregnancy, Childbirth and the Newborn* (Meadowbrook Press, Deephaven, Minnesota, 1984).

13. G. M. Stirrat, *Obstetrics* (Grant McIntyre, London, 1981).

14. Sally Inch, 'Management of the third stage of labour – another cascade of intervention?' *Midwifery*, I (1985), 114–22.

15. 'Should the cord be clamped?', *World Medicine*, 28 January, 1969.

16. Sally Inch, op. cit.

17. Frederick Leboyer, *Birth Without Violence* (Knopf, New York, 1976).

18. R. Rothenberg, 'Opthalmia neonatorum due to Neisseria gonorrhoeae', *Sexually Transmitted Diseases*, 6 (1979), 187–91.

Chapter 18: The Concept of Autonomy

1. Chapter title in Diana Korte and Roberta Scaer, *A Good Birth, A Safe Birth* (Bantam, New York, 1984).

PUBLICATIONS BY
SHEILA KITZINGER

The Experience of Childbirth: Gollancz, 1962; 5th Penguin edition, 1984. American, Dutch, Swedish, German, Italian and Portuguese editions.

Giving Birth: Gollancz, 1971. American edition.

Education and Counselling for Childbirth: Baillière Tindall, 1977. American, Belgian, Italian, German and Swedish editions.

Women as Mothers: Fontana, 1978. American, Swedish, Italian, German, Dutch and Portuguese editions.

The Place of Birth, ed. Sheila Kitzinger and John Davis, Oxford University Press, 1978.

Some Mothers' Experiences of Induced Labour: 2nd edition, National Childbirth Trust, 1978.

Birth at Home: Oxford University Press, 1979. American, German, Dutch, Swedish and Italian editions.

The Good Birth Guide: Fontana, 1979.

The New Good Birth Guide: Penguin, 1983.

The Experience of Breastfeeding: Penguin, 1984; revised edition, 1986. American, Polish, South African and German editions.

Pregnancy and Childbirth: Michael Joseph, 1980; Penguin, 1986. American, Brazilian, Danish, Dutch, Italian, Norwegian, Swedish, Portuguese, Spanish, Yugoslav, Afrikaans, Israeli, Australian, German, Finnish, Japanese editions.

Sheila Kitzinger's Birth Book: Fontana, 1981. German, American and Italian editions.

Some Women's Experiences of Episiotomy: with Rhiannon Walters, National Childbirth Trust, 1981.

Episiotomy: Physical and Emotional Aspects: ed. Sheila Kitzinger and Penny Simkin, National Childbirth Trust, 1981.

Episiotomy and the Second Stage of Labor: ed. Sheila Kitzinger and Penny Simkin, The Pennypress, Seattle, 1984; revised edition, 1986.

Birth over Thirty: Sheldon Press, 1982. Swedish, American, German, Dutch, Danish, Norwegian, Brazilian, Spanish and Yugoslav editions.

Women's Experience of Sex: Dorling Kindersley, 1983; Penguin, 1986. American, Australian, Danish, German, Dutch, Israeli, Norwegian, Finnish, Swedish, South African, Spanish, French and Brazilian editions.

Being Born: Dorling Kindersley, 1986. American, Australian, Canadian, Swedish, Japanese, Danish, Dutch, Finnish, Norwegian, Portuguese editions.

Celebration of Birth: The Pennypress, Seattle, 1986.

'What do women want?': chapter in *The Management of Labour*, ed. John Studd, Blackwells Scientific Publications, 1985.

'Episiotomy pain': chapter in *Textbook of Pain*, ed. Patrick D. Wall and Ronald Melzack, Churchill Livingstone, 1984.

'The social context of birth: some comparisons between childbirth in Jamaica and Britain': chapter in *Ethnography of Fertility and Birth*, ed. Carol P. MacCormack, Academic Press, 1982.

'The woman on the delivery table': chapter in *Woman on Woman*, ed. Margaret Laing, Sidgwick & Jackson, 1971.

'Experiences of obstetric practices in differing countries': chapter in *Pregnancy Care for the 1980s*, ed. Luke Zander and Geoffrey Chamberlain, Royal Society of Medicine, 1984.

Open University courses

Getting Ready for Pregnancy.

Understanding Pregnancy and Birth.

(Both from LMSO, Centre for Continuing Education, The Open University, PO Box 188, Milton Keynes MK3 6HW.)

USEFUL ADDRESSES

Acupuncture

British Acupuncture Association
and Register
34 Alderney Street
Westminster
London SW 1 V 4 EU
01-834 1012

AIDS and pregnancy

Healthline (confidential telephone
information service)
01-980 4848: 6–10 p.m.

Breastfeeding

La Leche League (Great Britain)
BM 3424
London WC 1 V 6 XX
01-404 5011

National Childbirth Trust
9 Queensborough Terrace
London W 2 3 TB
01-221 3833
*Can put you in touch with your local
branch.*

Caesarean birth

Caesarean Support Group of
Cambridge
42 Shelford Road
Cambridge
Cambridge 840561 or 841315

Greater Manchester Caesarean
Support Network
52 Ullswater Road
Tyldesly
Lancs. M 29 7 AQ
Atherton 873473

Childbirth organizations

Active Birth Centre
18 Laurier Road
London NW 5
01-267 3006

Association for Improvement in
Maternity Services (AIMS)
163 Liverpool Road
London N 1 ORF
01-278 5628

Birth Centre West London
7 Waldemar Avenue
London W 1 3
*They will also be able to give you
information about birth centres in
other parts of the country.*

National Childbirth Trust
9 Queensborough Terrace
London W 2 3 TB
01-221 3833
*Can put you in touch with your local
branch.*

The Maternity Alliance
59–61 Camden High Street
London NW 1 7 JL
01-388 6337

Complaints

Action for Victims of Medical
Accidents
121 Auckland Road
London SE 1

Patients' Association
Room 33
18 Charing Cross Road
London W C 2
01-240 0671
*Campaigning group for NHS patients.
Has information and advice on how to
make complaints.*

Death of a baby

The Compassionate Friends
25 Kingsdown Parade
Bristol
Bristol 47316

Foundation for the Study of Infant
  Deaths
23 St Peter's Square
London w6 9NW
01-748 7768

The Stillbirth Association
15a Christchurch Hill
London NW3 1JY
01-794 4601

Drugs

Drugs, Alcohol Nationally
01-250 3284

Drugwatch
157 Waterloo Road
London SE1 8XF
*Offers advice on all types of
  medication.*

Education about pregnancy and birth

Getting ready for pregnancy: study pack
  P901S (£12.00)
Pregnancy and birth: assessment pack
  P960A (£10.00)
Pregnancy and birth: video cassette
  VC9600 available for loan (£10
  for a six-week period) or purchase
  (£34.50)
Learning Materials Service
Centre for Continuing Education
Open University
PO Box 188
Milton Keynes MK3 6HW
0908 74066

Handicap

Association for Spina Bifida and
  Hydrocephalus
Tavistock House North
Tavistock Square
London WC1H 9HJ
01-388 1382

Child Crisis
Elizabeth Court
Fort Fareham Road
Fareham
Hampshire PO14 1DQ
0329 221530
*Support group for parents of sick and
  disabled children who have faced a
  life-or-death decision on their child's
  behalf.*

Contact a Family
16 Strutton Ground
London SW1P 2HP
*Links families with handicapped children
  into neighbourhood self-help groups.*

DIAL (Disablement Information and
  Advice Line)
Oxford 750190
*Free and confidential service of
  information and help for people with
  disabilities.*

Disabled Living Foundation
346 Kensington High Street
London W14
01-602 2491

The Down's Children's Association
4 Oxford Street
London W1N 9SL
01-580 0511

Family Services and Assessment
  Centre
16 Fitzroy Square
London W1P 5HQ
01-387 9571

HIPS (Help in Plaster and Splints)
22 Claudius Gardens
Chandlers Ford
Hants SO5 2NY
*Support group for parents of children
  with congenital displacement of the
  hips.*

Kith and Kids
58 The Avenue
Muswell Hill
London N10
01-883 8762
For parents of handicapped children.

National Association for Deaf Blind
and Rubella Handicapped
311 Gray's Inn Road
London WC1X 8PT
01-278 1000

National Society for Mentally
Handicapped Children
Pembridge Hall
17 Pembridge Square
London W2
01-229 8941

Parents' Lifeline
Station House
73d Stapleton Hall Road
London N4 3QF
01-263 2265
*Support group for parents of seriously ill
children in hospital*

Royal National Institute for the Blind
224 Great Portland Street
London W1N 6AA
01-388 1266

Royal National Institute for the Deaf
12a Rosebery Avenue
London EC1R 4TD
01-387 8033

Spastics Society
12 Park Crescent
London W1
01-636 5020

SPOD
8 Princess Road
Urmston
Manchester M31 3SS
*Support group for parents of children
with congenital abnormalities of the
lower limbs.*

Home birth

Independent Midwives' Association
65 Mount Nod Road
Streatham
London SW16 2LP

Society to Support Home
Confinements
17 Laburnum Avenue
Durham
0385 61325

Homeopathy

The British Homeopathic Association
27a Devonshire Street
London W1
01-953 2163

Hypnosis

British Society of Medical and Dental
Hypnotists
42 Links Road
Ashtead
Surrey KT21 2HJ

Midwives

Association of Radical Midwives
62 Greetby Hill
Ormskirk
Lancashire L39 2DT

Independent Midwives' Association
65 Mount Nod Road
Streatham
London SW16 2LP

Miscarriage

Miscarriage Association
18 Stoneybrook Close
West Bretton
Wakefield
West Yorkshire WF4 4TP
092-485 515

One-parent families

Gingerbread
35 Wellington Street
London WC2 7BN
01-240 0953/0954

The National Council for One-Parent
Families
255 Kentish Town Road
London NW5 2LX
01-267 1361

Postnatal problems

Association for Postnatal Illness
7 Gowan Avenue
Fulham
London SW6

MAMA (Meet a Mum Association)
26a Cumnor Hill
Oxford OX2 9HA

Pre-eclamptic toxaemia

Pre-Eclamptic Toxaemia Society
88 Plumberow
Lee Chapel North
Basildon
Essex SS15 5LQ

Premature babies

NIPPERS (National Information for
Parents of Prematures –
Education, Resources and
Support)
28 Swyncombe Avenue
London W5
01-847 4721

Scottish Premature Baby Support
Group
12 Corstorphine Hill Crescent
Edinburgh
031-334 1934

5 Boghead Road
Lenzie
Glasgow
041-777 6580

54 Grampian Way
Balloch
Eastfield
Cumbernauld

Psychotherapy

Women's therapy Centre
6 Manor Gardens
London N7 6LA
01-263 6200

Women's Counselling and Therapy
Service Ltd
Leeds 455725
*Covers Bradford/Leeds area and
offers individual counselling and
workshops.*

Relationship problems

The Institute of Marital Studies
Tavistock Centre
120 Belsize Lane
London NW3 5BA

Lesbian Line
01-251 6911
*Details of Lesbian mothers' groups all
over the country.*

London Marriage Guidance Council
76a New Cavendish Street
London W1
01-580 1087

Margaret Pyke Centre
27–35 Mortimer Street
London W1
01-580 3077
Help with sexual problems.

National Co-ordinating Committee of
Organisations for Parents Under
Stress
29 Newmarket Way
Hornchurch
Essex
Hornchurch 51538 (evenings)
*Can put you in touch with your local
Parents Anonymous branch.*

National Marriage Guidance Council
Herbert Gray College
Little Church Street
Rugby CV21 3AP

Westminster Pastoral Foundation
23 Kensington Square
London W8 5HN
01-937 6956

Sickle cell disease

Sickle Cell Society
c/o Brent Community Health
  Council
16 High Street
Harlesden NW 10 4LX
01-451 3293

Social Security

Free advice by phone: DHSS will
  pay for phone calls if you have
  social security queries. Dial 100,
  ask for Freephone DHSS, and you
  will be put through.

Women's Health Issues

Women's Health Information Centre
52–54 Featherstone Street
London EC 1
01-251 6580

Women's Reproductive Rights
  Information Centre
52–54 Featherstone Street
London EC 1
01-251 6332

Work outside the home

Nanny Sharing
44 Foresters Drive
Wallington
Surrey
01-647 7418

Working Mothers' Association
7 Spencer Walk
London SW 15 1PL
01-788 2565

Index